DEMENTIA AND HUMAN RIGHTS

Suzanne Cahill

P

First published in Great Britain in 2018 by

Policy Press
University of Bristol
1-9 Old Park Hill
Bristol
BS2 8BB
UK
t: +44 (0)117 954 5940
pp-info@bristol.ac.uk
www.policypress.co.uk

North America office:
Policy Press
c/o The University of Chicago Press
1427 East 60th Street
Chicago, IL 60637, USA
t: +1 773 702 7700
f: +1 773-702-9756
sales@press.uchicago.edu
www.press.uchicago.edu

British Library Cataloguing in Publication Data
A catalogue record for this book is available from the British Library

Library of Congress Cataloging-in-Publication Data
A catalog record for this book has been requested

ISBN 978-1-4473-3140-7 paperback
ISBN 978-1-4473-3137-7 hardcover
ISBN 978-1-4473-3141-4 ePub
ISBN 978-1-4473-3142-1 Mobi
ISBN 978-1-4473-3138-4 epdf

Cover design by Qube Design Associates, Bristol
Front cover image: Getty

I would like to dedicate this book to:

Alph O'Connor and Benny O'Connor and

to all people who have dementia and their

family members.

Contents

List of tables and figures

Tables

Figures

Acknowledgements

This book could not have been written without the support of a number of colleagues, friends and relatives to whom I am very grateful. First my thanks are due to Professor Bernard Walsh, Dr Declan Byrne, Carol Murphy and Lorcan Birthistle from St James's Hospital, Dublin, for their belief and confidence in the feasibility of this book and for their supporting me to take time off work to write it. During that eight-month period, Matthew Gibb took over from me, as Director at the Dementia Services Information and Development Centre (DSIDC), and I owe Matthew a special debt of gratitude. I also wish to thank Professor Davis Coakley and Professor Brian Lawlor (founders of the DSIDC) for the continuous support shown to me throughout my lengthy and very fulfilling career there as Director.

Prior to setting out on this project, I knew little about human rights, and I found in a friend and colleague Dr Hasheem Mannan (University College Dublin) much inspiration. I would like to thank Hasheem for his gently ushering me into the complex area of the human rights literature and his early most valuable advice. A big thank you is also due to Dr Edurne García Iriarte for teaching me all I currently know about 'disabilities studies' and for allowing me to share my embryonic thoughts on 'dementia as a disability' with her Master's in Disability students at Trinity College Dublin. At Trinity College, I would also like to acknowledge the support, encouragement and advice given to me by Professor Robbie Gilligan, Professor Desmond O'Neill and Professor Virpi Timonen.

The voice and perspective of the individual living with dementia was central to this book, and in this context I particularly want to thank Helen Rochford Brennan, Chairperson of the Irish and European Working Group on Dementia, for her support and contribution. I would also like to acknowledge the support offered to me by Professor Peter Mittler.

Whilst researching and writing the book, Dr Emer Begley and Avril Easton, both former students of mine employed at The Alzheimer Society of Ireland, gave generously of their time, for which I am very grateful. Gráinne McGettrick, former Policy Officer at The Alzheimer Society, was the person who first inspired me to apply the human rights lens to framing dementia, and I would like to thank Gráinne for her insights and earlier helpful discussions. At Alzheimer Europe, I would especially like to acknowledge and thank Dr Ana Diaz-Ponce for her generosity and support: Ana has always been such a ray of sunshine in my life and continues to be hugely missed by me as I know by many others in the dementia field in Ireland. At Alzheimer Europe, my thanks are also due to Dr Dianne Gove.

Across the world, there are many other experts in the field of dementia studies who have supported me over recent months. In no particular order these include Professor Mary Marshall, Professor Sube Banerjee, Professor Linda Clare, Professor John Keady, Professor Øyvind Kirkevold, Professor Steve Iliffe, Professor Bob Woods, Professor Louise Robinson, Dr Torhild Holthe, Dr Fiona Kelly, Glenn Rees, Marc Wortmann, Marie Jo Guisset, Sue Benson and Marianne Schulz. Much of my critical thinking about dementia occurred during the period I was establishing the Living with Dementia postgraduate research programme at Trinity College, through a research grant awarded to me by The Atlantic Philanthropies and at Atlantic, I would especially like to thank Mary Sutton, Ken Logue, Tom Costello and Julie Browne for their confidence in me and support of my effort.

Several friends and close colleagues from Ireland provided helpful feedback on earlier draft chapters of this book. In this context I would like to thank Professor Eamon O'Shea, Dr Maria Pierce, Dr Tony Foley, Dr Emer Begley, Dr Sarah Donnelly, Dr Fíona Kelly, Dr Jackie Eustace, Daphne Stephenson and Athina Georgantzi. More than anyone else I must acknowledge a great debt to Professor Margaret Shapiro, my former PhD supervisor and close friend, who has kept my thinking sharp and has read and provided valuable feedback to me on every chapter of the book. There are several other colleagues, friends and former students whose insights over the years have greatly enriched this book and whose works I have attempted to thread through some of the chapters and to whom I am very grateful. These include Dr Treena Parsons, Dr Andrew Bobersky, Professor Kate Irving and Dr Sabina Brennan.

My friends near and far in Ireland, Sweden and Australia likewise need to be acknowledged. In Jönköping (my second home), special thanks are due to Arja and Bernt Ringström, two wonderful friends and neighbours. Arja, it so happens, is a nurse practitioner who works in a specialist dementia care unit. She has opened up so many opportunities for me to learn all I currently know about the Swedish health and social care system for older people. My thanks are due also to my family in Ireland present and past who have given me so much, especially my sisters Jackie and Michele and their families, my cousin Derek O'Connor and my new family in Sweden, especially Rigmor, Olle and Carl. Susie Cox is a wonderful friend to whom I am so grateful for her proofreading the entire book. A special thanks to Policy Press, particularly Isabel Bainton and Rebecca Tomlinson for their endless patience with me throughout and to Ruth Wallace for her editorial wisdom and amazing skill in helping me structure the final version of this manuscript. Finally, the greatest acknowledgement in this work rests with my husband Thomas, whose love, support, encouragement, patience, technical help and confidence in me throughout the time spent researching and writing this book has been so utterly amazing – Jag vet att jag inte kunde ha gjort detta utan ditt stöd!

Foreword

For most of the past century, people with dementia were viewed through a biomedical lens and treated accordingly. This was logical to a degree because dementia is a syndrome produced by many different diseases that damage the brain and it is true that dementia is defined by dysfunctions in particular aspects of explicit memory, language, visual perception, and the organization of movement as demonstrated on standard neuropsychological tests. The use of a biomedical lens alone, however, is inappropriate if one seeks to understand the subjective experience and remaining abilities of people living with dementia.

In the past thirty years, through the increased use of a biopsychosocial lens, we have learned that the actions of people living with dementia are not due solely to brain damage, but also involve (1) their psychological reactions to the effects of brain damage, (2) how they are treated in social situations, and (3) their reactions to said treatment. We have learned also that people with dementia are semiotic subjects: they can act intentionally and appropriately in response to the meaning of social situations. As well, they are able to evaluate those situations in terms of the values and meanings they have held dear for the balance of their adult lives. For example, they can respond appropriately to the emotional needs of others, seek to avoid potentially embarrassing and humiliating situations, feel and demonstrate self-respect and proper pride, feel and demonstrate loneliness as well as being loved and respected, miss their loved ones, express themselves creatively, appreciate and display humour, along with a host of other healthy socio-cognitive abilities. People living with dementia share much social and emotional common ground with people who are deemed healthy. This has become increasingly apparent as their voices have been heard and respected as meaningful rather than being summarily dismissed as reflections of pathology and as they have been engaged in places other than hospital and memory clinics. Indeed, although a person with dementia may have difficulty finding and pronouncing words and organizing them syntactically, if we assume that the person is trying to tell us something meaningful, it is possible to facilitate the person's expression of his or her thoughts and open lines of communication.

Our increased understanding of the remaining strengths possessed by people with dementia requires that we attend ever more carefully to how they are treated with respect to their rights as human beings and the obligations and duties of those deemed healthy when interacting with them. All too often, people with dementia are unintentionally treated in depersonalizing ways that Tom Kitwood described as 'malignant social psychology', that attack their feelings of self-worth. If misunderstood, a diagnosis of dementia can lead to a person being stripped of the right to be treated with the same respect and care and the same legal rights that that person enjoyed years before – indeed, the day before – he or she was diagnosed. Should a person with dementia lose the right to make decisions about important matters in his or her life? What criteria should be used to support some kind of limitation on decision-making and what sorts of treatment ought to be sanctioned or disallowed? What 'top-down' governmental legal steps ought to be taken with the input of people with dementia to protect their human rights and improve their care? What sorts of 'bottom up' educational efforts should be undertaken to provide people in the everyday social world with an informed understanding of the cognitive strengths possessed by people diagnosed so as to supplant the stereotyped negative version presented so often in the mass media? Would treating dementia as a disability provide people diagnosed with fundamental human rights as understood by the World Health Organization and the UN Convention on Rights of Persons with Disabilities?

These are a few of the extremely important, complex nuanced matters that Suzanne Cahill addresses from a policy and practice perspective in *Dementia and human rights*. One of the central ideas in the book is that the voices of people with dementia must be heard, honoured, facilitated, and supported. This is altogether appropriate especially if their rights and privileges regarding their treatment and decision-making ability are at stake. The fact that a person has dementia according to standard tests of cognitive function may have little to nothing to do with his or her ability to choose not to have a colostomy operation, for example. It is quite possible, at least in the United States, for someone to obtain the legal right, via plenary guardianship, to force a person with dementia to have such an operation against his or her will. This is but one example of any number of ways in which the rights of people with dementia can be summarily abrogated.

How a society treats its most vulnerable members clearly reflects that society's character. A 'right' is something that requires no justification. People possess human rights as a matter of definition. People living with dementia have not, as a result of their diagnosis, lost their humanity or their human rights unless those of us deemed healthy decide to strip that humanity and those rights from them, in which case dementia alone is not to blame.

It is rather easy for me to say all this. The case must be made far more deliberately, logically, and legally, and that is what Suzanne Cahill has done by applying a human rights lens and drawing on supporting evidence in this important book that is not really about 'them' who are diagnosed with dementia, but truly about all of us and the shared humanity that is ours to keep and respect or to lose.

Steven R. Sabat, PhD
Professor Emeritus of Psychology
Georgetown University
Washington, DC

PART ONE

A conceptual framework

ONE

An introduction to human rights and dementia

Introduction

"The rights and needs of persons with dementia have been given low priority in the national and global agenda. In particular, with the progression of the disease, as their autonomy decreases, persons with dementia tend to be isolated, excluded and subject to abuse and violence", so said Ms Rosa Kornfeld-Matte, UN Independent Expert on the Enjoyment of All Human Rights by Older People, on the opening day of the first Ministerial Conference on Global Action against Dementia held in Geneva in March 2015.

Ms Kornfeld-Matte went on to say how it was critical to tackle dementia through a human rights-based perspective because people with dementia are 'rights holders', and because states and other stakeholders are 'duty bearers'. According to her, policies, legislation, regulations, institutions and budgets relating to dementia should all be embedded in a system of rights and obligations. She concluded this powerful statement with the following provocative appeal:

> I call on all States and other stakeholders to adopt a human rights-based approach when addressing dementia. Dementia is a public health issue, but also a human rights concern. Persons with dementia should be able to enjoy their rights and fundamental freedoms in any circumstances. Their dignity, beliefs, needs and privacy must be respected at all stages of the disease. (Rosa Kornfeld-Matte, 2015)

Later during the same conference, two personal appeals to have their human rights respected were made by young people: Kate Swaffer, an Australian nurse, author, co-founder, Chair and CEO of Dementia Alliance International (DAI), and Chair of Alzheimer's Australia Dementia Advisory Group, who was first diagnosed with dementia at the age of 49, and Mike Ellenbogen, an American IT executive, who first presented with symptoms of dementia at the age of 39, and a decade later was finally diagnosed.

In an audience of some 450 people representing 89 countries around the world, both Kate and Mike discussed the many challenges including discriminatory practices they have encountered as a direct result of having dementia. These include: their efforts to obtain a diagnosis, to live a life like others and 'not be shut away', to continue to drive, work, manage their finances, access services and be treated with dignity and respect. They appealed for the human rights of people living with dementia to be protected, for a more balanced research agenda to be developed with an equal focus on care and cure, and for more ethical integrated care pathways, including, in Kate's case, rehabilitation services to be made available. Through their thought-provoking contributions including lived experiences, they reminded this large international audience of the marginalization, social exclusion, indignities and injustices people with dementia often experience.

The conference was unique since it was the first of its kind where the World Health Organization (WHO) brought together individuals living with dementia, their family members, government ministers, clinicians, researchers, service planners, service providers and dementia advocacy groups, including Alzheimer Europe and other national Alzheimer societies and associations, to collectively adopt a human rights-based approach to dementia, a perspective later incorporated by Dr Margaret Chan, WHO's CEO, when, in her concluding remarks and final call for action, she proclaimed:

> We [the participants] call for actions ... raising the priority accorded to global efforts to tackle dementia ... strengthening capacity, leadership, governance, multisectoral action and partnerships to accelerate responses to address dementia; promoting a better understanding of dementia, raising public awareness and engagement, *including respect for the human rights* of people living with dementia, reducing stigma and discrimination, and fostering greater participation, social inclusion and integration... (Dr Margaret Chan, quoted in WHO, 2015b, p 43; emphasis added)

That was March 2015, and since then, a slowly evolving rights-based dementia movement has begun to gain traction across the world through the work of the WHO, Alzheimer's Disease International (ADI), Alzheimer Europe, DAI, the Dementia Engagement &

Empowerment Project (DEEP), the Scottish Dementia Working Group (SDWG), the Irish Dementia Working Group (IDWG), and several other regional and national dementia working and advisory groups. Although calls for the expansion of this rights-based dementia movement have recently been made (Mental Health Foundation, 2015; Rees, 2015; WHO, 2015a; Williamson, 2015; DAI, 2016; Hare, 2016; Swaffer, 2016, Shakespeare et al, 2017), curiously, a rights-based approach, reflecting a broader emphasis on autonomy, empowerment, dignity, social inclusion, participation and non-discrimination, with some few exceptions, has not as yet been explicitly applied to most countries' policy responses and dementia service developments.

It is timely therefore to move the policy debate forward, given the fact that dementia can significantly compromise an individual's ability to protect their own human rights (Kelly and Innes, 2012; Hare, 2016), those living with the condition are often marginalized and stigmatized (Innes et al, 2004; Bartlett and O'Connor, 2007; ADI, 2012), and virtually every aspect of dementia practice, policy and research (WHO, 2015a), from diagnosis to death, lends itself well to a critical analysis from a human rights-based perspective.

Rationale for writing this book

That first ministerial global conference in 2015, which I was fortunate to attend, along with the inspirational paper on human rights and dementia delivered by my Irish colleague, Gráinne McGettrick, at the Alzheimer Europe conference in Glasgow in 2014, combined with my own professional experience working in the field, a career straddling two continents and three decades, has more recently set me thinking critically about dementia as a human rights issue, and has planted the seeds for writing this book. And certainly the dementia landscape and the theoretical frameworks used by me now to understand, research and teach dementia courses have changed significantly since the late 1980s, when I first became employed in the field in Australia.

Indeed, my first real exposure to what was to become a lifetime career working in the area of dementia was 30 years ago (1988), when employed at the University of Queensland, I had responsibility for coordinating a longitudinal study of 'family caregivers'. That study investigated the economic, emotional and social costs of Alzheimer's disease (Rosenman and Cahill, 1989; Cahill and Rosenman, 1991). This was the era when Alzheimer's disease, called at the time 'Senile Dementia of the Alzheimer Type' (SDAT), was viewed almost exclusively through a biomedical lens – framed as a cognitive brain disorder – and when the disease model remained largely unchallenged. It was an era when concepts such as personhood, selfhood, social citizenship, autonomy, self-determination and human rights had not as yet come to the fore: in short, it was an era of therapeutic nihilism, 'When [once] psychiatry had made a probable diagnosis … its task was virtually complete…' (Kitwood, 1993a, p 541), and when caregivers were seen as the hidden victims (Holicky, 1996) of an illness that robbed individuals' of their minds and resulted in never-ending funerals (van Gorp and Vercruysse, 2012).

In keeping with the scope of much social science research on dementia at the time, that study was largely quantitative: its primary focus was on caregiver burden, dementia severity, the cost of care, time from diagnosis to nursing home placement and so on. 'Family caregivers' were the unit of analysis, and from a research perspective, it would have been unheard of then to interview the individual or attempt to investigate the subjective experience of a person living with dementia.

Several years later, whilst doing the fieldwork for my PhD (Cahill, 1997), another longitudinal study that explored the gendered politics of caregiving and particularly factors associated with starting and stopping the 'caring role', I had the privilege of spending much time again in the homes of people diagnosed with dementia, conducting in-depth interviews with 'family caregivers' about service needs and service use. The interview data collected was often raw and challenging, and I remember at times being struck by its rich content: the strong gendered kinship obligations to sustain caring roles, despite a loved one's extraordinarily high dependency needs, the ploys used by some people, generally women, to reduce the distressing effects of the 'behavioural and psychological symptoms of dementia' including aggression, paranoia, repetitive questioning, sleep disturbance and delusions, and, at the heart of it, the love, humanity and compassion many family members expressed for their relatives.

But other chilling memories from the fieldwork for that study remain etched in my memory. These include detailed narratives told to me by family members, often in the presence of a loved one, which sadly honed in on their at times irresponsible and embarrassing behaviour, often with a distinct lack of regard for the impact their storytelling had on their relative sitting next to them. It was as if they assumed that the person was sub-human, no longer existed, and because of the dementia could no longer experience humiliation. On a few occasions I remember trying to quickly change the subject, that we move to another room, or that we talk about these issues later, but to no avail.

A common response was, "Oh don't worry, she doesn't understand anything now anyway." And not surprisingly, there were times when I left these interviews, feeling I had behaved unethically and concerned about the impact these narratives had on the individual experiencing the symptoms. We can never assume that a person diagnosed with dementia lacks insight or is unaware (Howorth and Saper, 2003).

Later, as Director of the Dementia Services Information and Development Centre (DSIDC) in Ireland, I had exposure to accounts of indignities and the neglect of the individuals' human rights, through some of the narratives told to me during training days, and through my own personal observations at the nursing homes where these workshops took place. Examples include nursing home residents with no next of kin at times dressed in communal gowns; individuals with severe dementia essentially warehoused, sitting motionless in Buxton chairs and locked away in large Nightingale wards (with no subdivisions) and with no evidence of any psychosocial stimulation. Other examples include the lack of respect for residents' privacy rights and their occasionally being referred to by busy inexperienced staff as "another Alzheimer's".

Likewise as a Lecturer in Trinity College Dublin and through students' Master's and PhD dissertations, more subtle examples of human rights breaches were brought to my attention. These include the massive imbalance of power relations in hospitals, where at care planning meetings, supposedly organized to empower the 'patient' and family members, the professional voice often dominated, and where 'patients' with a cognitive impairment were at risk of being talked over by health service professionals who sometimes referred to them in the third person (Donnelly, 2012). Other examples include reminiscence work being conducted in noisy sub-optimal physical environments, facilitated by staff, inexperienced and untrained in reminiscence (Parsons, 2015), and the lack of choice in long-term care facilities available to people living with dementia, especially the absence of 'housing with care' models (Convery, 2014).

It is important to create a balanced picture, and whilst this book is concerned with the neglect and at the extreme violation of human rights of the individual living with dementia, it needs to be highlighted that over the years I have worked in Australia and in Ireland with many exceptionally dedicated practitioners whose commitment to the individual diagnosed with dementia has been beyond the call of duty. I have also had the opportunity to visit many day care centres, nursing homes and community hospitals, where staffs' understanding of personhood, social citizenship and person-centred care practices has been second to none. Being Irish, several of the examples drawn on in the book come from Ireland, but this is not to suggest that the quality of dementia services in Ireland is in any way inferior to services delivered in other European countries and elsewhere.

In fact, I hold a vivid recollection of many years ago, visiting a care home in a Nordic country, which will remain nameless. During the visit with colleagues VT and JC from Trinity College Dublin, as we were about to leave a state-of-the-art dementia unit, where on entry we had been welcomed with the delightful sights of residents and staff dancing to music, I heard some scratching on a door. Curious, I asked the Director of Nursing to investigate what was going on. She then produced keys and in front of all three of us, she opened the door and released four residents, each of whom had been deliberately locked away during our visit. One of these ladies had soiled herself whilst locked inside the same room, or who knows, perhaps this was the reason she had been locked in during our visit. However, what I do recall is the undignified and insensitive manner in which the incident was managed, as in front of all three of us, strangers in her home, the Director lifted the lady's skirt and commented disapprovingly on the incident.

These, along with other similar incidents, have convinced me that the individual living with dementia is exceptionally vulnerable and is at a heightened risk of having their human rights violated (WHO, 2015a; Hare, 2016). A human rights lens provides a very useful tool to rethink and realign dementia policy and practice (Mental Health Foundation, 2015), yet often practitioners and policy-makers are not thinking about human rights issues when supporting a person with dementia (Forbat, 2006; Kelly and Innes, 2012). There is a gap in our understanding of dementia from a social justice perspective, and an urgent need to interrogate dementia using a human rights lens.

Aims and objectives

This book therefore attempts to address this gap in understanding. Throughout the chapters I argue that dementia is a disability, and that because of this, the individual just like any person with a disability is entitled to each of the rights set out in the UN's *Convention on the Rights of Persons with Disabilities (CRPD)* (UN, 2006) (hereafter referred to only as CRPD). By operationalizing a selection of these rights, the book provides a fresh conceptual lens to interrogate dementia policy and practice. Throughout the chapters and wherever possible, the reader will gain new insights into the way a cognitively impaired person constructs their own reality, how that person makes sense of their world, and how the individual is responded to through current health and social care policies.

The main aim of the book is to challenge thinking, provoke debate and demonstrate how a human rights-based approach, underpinned by the social model of disability, transports dementia into a new and exciting arena (McGettrick, 2014; Mental Health Foundation, 2015). This book brings to the fore critical issues relating to disability, human rights, social justice, discrimination, oppression, equality and participation. Within the chapters, new analytical tools are introduced that can be used to interrogate and deconstruct dementia, thereby further expanding the dementia policy and practice debate.

A central and unifying theme underpinning each chapter is recognition of the civil, political, social, economic and cultural rights the individual living with dementia possesses, to live well, free from stigma and discrimination, to engage in decision-making on matters directly relevant to their lives, to have choice, exercise autonomy and where necessary, to receive support to do so, and to be valued and treated with dignity and respect. It is argued that to achieve this, the voice of the person with dementia must be heard, service providers must be upskilled, public policy must be reframed and an intersectoral approach needs to be adopted whereby change at an international level is driven by strong political leadership. In this way, the book provides a timely framework in which to expand knowledge and understanding of dementia, incorporating into analysis key concepts including personhood, autonomy, participation, equality, solidarity and human rights.

Policy-makers, researchers, health service professionals and care staff, along with students in medicine, nursing, occupational therapy, physiotherapy, psychiatry, psychology, social work, gerontology and disability studies, will gain new insights from this book that builds on earlier critical perspectives (see Kitwood, 1990, 1993a, b, 1995, 1997a, b; Sabat, 1994, 2001, 2005, 2011; Marshall, 1998, 1999, 2001, 2003, 2005; Innes et al, 2004; Bartlett and O'Connor, 2007, 2010; Hughes, 2011, 2014). The book will also be of interest to people living with dementia, their family members and their advocates. It seeks to improve policy and practice responses by arguing that the individual living with dementia has a disability in keeping with the CRPD's description of disability (Mittler, 2015), and therefore that person has full entitlement to all the rights set out in the CRPD. Original insights are proposed as to how a rights-based approach to dementia can be applied in practice and incorporated into policy development.

Throughout the chapters it will be contended that rights-based initiatives, embodying human rights principles and standards, can ignite change in dementia policy and practice (McGettrick, 2014), and can improve quality of life and quality of care for all those affected by this condition. A rights-based approach has the potential to bring about a seismic shift in thinking (Quinn, 2010) as it demands accountability, dignity, fairness and social action. A rights-based approach challenges power relations, changes negative discourse, helps create a new vision, and turns paternalistic approaches to dementia on their head. In short, a rights-based approach results in a levelling of the playing field, bringing the person with dementia to the centre stage and listening to the individual and collective voice (McGettrick, 2014).

However, before proceeding to outline the conceptual framework to be used in the book, it is first necessary to define what is meant by 'human rights', and to briefly review the relevant documents, including declarations, covenants and treaties, relating to human rights, especially the *Universal Declaration of Human Rights* (UDHR) (UN, 1948). Many diverse definitions of 'human rights' exist and 'countless pages have been written on the idea of human rights' (Tobin, 2012, p 50). In the section to follow, the focus is on attempting to simplify the concept of human rights by providing the reader with a broad overview as an introduction to the topic (Clapham, 2007).

Defining and describing 'human rights'

Numerous definitions of human rights exist, but an easy and helpful definition is one provided by the UK's Equality and Human Rights Commission (EHRC, 2010, p 6), which states that:

> Human rights are a set of basic rights and freedoms that everyone is entitled to, regardless of who they are. They are about how the State must treat you. They recognize that everyone is of equal value, has the right to make their own decisions and should be treated with fairness, dignity and respect. Human rights have been written down in international agreements such as the Universal Declaration of Human Rights (1948) and the European Convention on Human Rights (1950).

Missing from this definition, is the fact that human rights are also about how people (not just governments) treat other people and how human rights connect all of us to each other through shared rights and responsibilities (AHRC, 2014). They were first legally defined by international agreement, after the horrors of the Second World War, and since then many different treaties/agreements pertaining to human rights have been established (BIHR, 2010). They cover virtually every aspect of human activity and can be classified as civil, political, economic, social and cultural. Human rights are an important part of how people and societies interact in family life, in the community, at schools and at work, in politics and in international relations (AHRC, 2014). Examples include civil and political rights such as the right to life, to liberty, privacy and freedom from torture, and social, economic and cultural rights such as the right to health, education, to an adequate standard of living and to participate in cultural life, recreation, leisure and sport. A key difference between the two sets of rights is that in the case of civil and political rights, governments must ensure that they and others are not denying people access to these rights, whereas in the context of economic, social and cultural rights, governments are obliged to be proactive and take action to ensure that these rights are fulfilled (AHRC, 2014).

Human rights are universal (apply to everyone), indivisible (have equal status and cannot be placed in hierarchical order), inalienable (cannot be given or removed) and inabrogable (cannot be voluntarily relinquished or traded for other privileges) (Clapham, 2007; Ife, 2012). They are based on principles of fairness, equality, dignity and respect, and are about how people and public authorities treat individuals. Human rights are also reciprocal, meaning that people have both rights and responsibilities, and nations and people are both rights bearers and duty holders (Tobin, 2012).

Marks (2014) notes that human rights straddle both philosophical (ordinary rights) and legal discourse. In law, for example, rights refer to any entitlement that is legally protected, whilst in philosophical discussions, rights refer to entitlements associated with being human or being a citizen (Marks, 2014). Human rights can be *absolute*, which means that they can never be restricted, as, for example, the right to life. They can be *limited*, which means that rights can have boundaries in very defined circumstances as, for example, if a person has a mental health problem (BIHR, 2010). Rights can also be *qualified*, which means that in the interest of proportionality and to protect the rights of others, they may be restricted (Hughes, 2010).

Whilst throughout history human rights principles such as ethics, justice, non-discrimination and dignity have been very important in developing human societies (AHRC, 2014), it was the atrocities and violations that occurred during the Second World War that garnered global opinion that such massive destruction of people should never recur and in an effort to create a more peaceful world, the *Universal Declaration of Human Rights* (UDHR) (UN, 1948) was launched (for a more detailed account of the history of human rights, see Forsythe et al, 2006; Alston and Megret, 2008). The UDHR was the first global, explicit commitment to the fact that human rights were considered an essential entitlement to all human beings internationally. At the time, it was considered revolutionary, as instead of nations having responsibility for their own citizens, all nations would now be ruled by principles and laws, and would have to comply with minimum standards set down by the United Nations (UN) (Reichert, 2011). Although not legally binding, the UDHR is said to provide the most authoritative statement on international human rights norms (Donnelly, 2007).

Negative and positive rights

In everyday language, human rights are referred to as negative or positive (Gauri and Gloppin, 2012; Velasquez et al, 2014). Negative rights, also known as natural rights or civil and political rights, require protection against abuse and include the right to freedom from discrimination to free expression and to privacy. These rights are negative since they permit the rights holder to prevent others from interfering in their lives (Velasquez et al, 2014). The right to privacy, for example, places a claim on others not to intrude or interfere with one's private activities. Negative rights have tended to dominate global understandings of human rights, leading to the dominance of the law as a human rights profession (Ife, 2012). In the UDHR, by far the majority of rights (Articles 3-21) refer to negative rights.

By contrast, positive rights require not just protection but also realization and fulfilment by way of government intervention or private provision. These rights are positive since they place a claim on others for positive assistance to enable rights to be fulfilled (Velasquez et al, 2014). Examples include the right to healthcare, education and social security. Respecting a positive right requires more than non-interference, since it places an obligation on others to help maintain the welfare/wellbeing of those in need (Velasquez et al, 2014). In the context of people living with dementia, both their negative and positive rights need consideration, as does the level or degree of realization of all human rights, from non-fulfilment to generous fulfilment (Townsend, 2006).

Human rights declarations and covenants

Earlier reference was made to the UDHR (UN, 1948) and within two years of its launch the *European Convention on Human Rights* (ECHR) was drafted. The ECHR is an agreement within Europe, established between 47 member states, and commits these states to protect their citizens' fundamental freedoms and human rights. It is said to be the European version or classification of the rights set out in the UDHR (UN, 1948), and decrees that all legislation, government policy and those of public authorities must comply with the ECHR (Mental Health Foundation, 2015). Countries that sign up to the ECHR and fail to respect the rights it espouses are breaking international law (BIHR, 2010). There are several other covenants and treaties concerning people's human rights, the most important of which are the 1966 International Covenant on Civil and Political Rights and the International Covenant on Economic, Social and Cultural rights, which, together with the UDHR, form the International Bill of Human Rights.

In this book, the chosen compass for the analysis of human rights is the CRPD, although the UDHR is important since it has shaped and informed the CRPD, and is said to be at the centre of demands made by people globally for their rights to be respected and protected (Clapham, 2007). The UDHR has also been explicitly referred to by WHO (2015a); in the context of advocating for all dementia-related policy, practice and research to be underpinned by rights-based principles, when it states:

> All measures related to dementia adopted by States and other stakeholders should be linked to human rights standards contained in, and principles derived from, the *Universal Declaration of Human Rights* and other international human rights instruments. This includes all measures adopted related to dementia, including the development of policies and legislation, the implementation, monitoring and evaluation system and the entire care chain, from raising awareness to prevention, diagnosis, care and services and research programmes. (WHO, 2015a, p 4)

The UDHR remains the international human rights document with the greatest moral force (Ife, 2012). It has provided a strong foundation for a number of other covenants, treaties and declarations pertaining to human rights (Reichert, 2011). Many of the Articles in the UDHR address similar topics to those contained in the CRPD, and a selection of these Articles are critically reviewed in later chapters of this book, but first, to a broader discussion about the classification of human rights and a distinction between rights and needs.

Dementia as a human rights issue: a distinction between rights and needs

Although throughout this book dementia is conceptualized as a disability (see Chapter Two), as a disability, dementia is also a human rights issue (WHO and The World Bank, 2011) since, as stated earlier, the individual diagnosed is at heightened risk of experiencing injustices, marginalization and discrimination (Bartlett and O'Connor, 2010; ADI, 2012, Mittler, 2015; WHO, 2015a; Hare, 2016). It is not uncommon for a person living with dementia to encounter structural barriers, as, for example, attempting to access diagnostic and post-diagnostic services (Begley, 2009; Boyle, 2010; Bobersky, 2013; Donnelly et al, 2016; Swaffer, 2016). A person may also be subjected to attitudinal barriers such as stigma and prejudice (Bartlett, 2000; Cahill et al, 2006; Gove et al, 2015; Hare, 2016), their autonomy rights may be overlooked (Boyle, 2008; O'Connor and Purves, 2009), and respect for their dignity and privacy may also be disregarded (Manthorpe et al, 2010; UNECE, 2015b).

In recasting dementia as a human rights issue it is also important to consider human needs. Whilst rights are statements of facts, which allow an individual to place a lawful claim on others, needs are 'statements of values, of ideologies rather than statements of fact' (Ife, 2012, p 126). The word 'need' conjures up a notion of a vague deficit, that something is required for an outcome to be achieved (Ife, 2012). Accordingly, needs are subjective and relative (Bradshaw, 1994) and appeal to charity, whereas rights are objective and absolute, and require legal or political intervention. Stated simply, a human rights approach translates the notion of needs into a matter of entitlement with dignity (Solis, 2014).

A further fundamental difference between needs and rights is that human needs are generally hierarchical and can be prioritized, whereas rights are indivisible (Ife, 2012). As noted by Ife (2012), Maslow's hierarchy of needs (1970) provides a useful example of how human needs can be classified from basic/fundamental needs to higher-level needs including belongingness, love, esteem and self-actualization. In his earlier writings, Bradshaw (1972) developed a typology of needs that he referred to as (i) normative – expert-defined needs; (ii) felt needs – subjective wants; (iii) expressed needs such as demands; and (iv) comparative needs, meaning the comparison of levels of provision of groups or areas (Bradshaw, 1972). In Bradshaw's typology, *expressed needs* are probably most closely aligned with human rights.

Kitwood's cluster of needs

Kitwood, whose contribution to the field of dementia studies has been enormous and whose works (Kitwood, 1990, 1993a, b, 1995, 1997a, b) will be drawn on in later chapters of this book, highlighted five main psychological needs experienced by people living with dementia, namely, the need for comfort, attachment, identity, occupation and activity (Kitwood, 1997b). In his seminal book (Kitwood, 1997a), where he deconstructs dementia, Kitwood claims that each of these needs is subsumed under a fundamental need we all share for love: 'it might be said that there is only one all-encompassing need – for love' (Kitwood, 1997a, p 81). He argues that in practice, failure to address these five psychological needs can result in the erosion of 'personhood', an important concept, defined by him as a 'status that is bestowed upon one human being, by others, in the context of relationship and social being. It implies recognition, respect and trust' (Kitwood, 1997a, p 8).

In his theorizing about dementia, Kitwood points to the importance of interpersonal relations as a critical component of the subjective experience of dementia. He asserts that many of the behaviours exhibited by people diagnosed with dementia are often attributed to their diseased brain without any consideration given to the social context in which the behaviour occurs or the everyday real-life situations of the individual (Kitwood, 1993a). He believed it was incompetent to regard the 'problem' of dementia as being solely related to the neurological impairment, as each and everyone of us in close contact with the person was part of the 'problem' by virtue of our attitudes, beliefs, assumptions and behaviours (Kitwood, 1993a).

Whilst volumes have been written about Kitwood's work since his premature death, and whilst his writings have inspired great critical thinking, Kitwood's theorizing has also been heavily critiqued (see, for example, Adams, 1996; Baldwin and Capstick, 2007; Dewing, 2008). My own criticism of Kitwood's work is based on the reductionist approach he adopted, and his readiness to point to interpersonal relations as being critical components of the experience of dementia and to ignore socio-political structures. In other words, his overall analysis was apolitical (Bartlett and O'Connor, 2010). He claimed that the neglect of people's psychological *needs* contributed to their ill-being by undermining personhood. However, he failed to elevate these *needs* to *rights* and point to the failure of political structures and social systems to respect, protect and fulfil people's rights.

Bartlett and O'Connor (2007) argue that the citizenship/rights lens has a political dimension absent from personhood, making it a more effective frame for achieving social and political changes. I would contend that had Kitwood reframed *needs*/deficits as *rights*, as, for example, the right to privacy, dignity, recreation, independence and to be protected from cruel, inhuman or degrading treatment or punishment, this rights-based approach would have provided a much stronger moral framework for political redress in the area of dementia, including the necessary policy and legislative changes. In other words, Kitwood could have pushed the boundaries further, by arguing for the regulation of personhood, through legal reform and through the granting of legal capacity to people who had a cognitive impairment (Quinn, 2010; Flynn and Arstein-Kerslake, 2014). This would have advanced personhood more positively, by opening up opportunities of personal freedom for the individual diagnosed. Instead Kitwood framed psychological needs as 'soft rights' (Mental Health Foundation, 2015). This meant that deficits or needs were constructed as personal rather than political, analysed at a micro rather than macro level, and addressed by pointing to solutions found at an interpersonal rather than socio-political structural level.

Treating people as sub-human or non-persons

Earlier in this chapter, reference was made to the atrocities experienced by certain individuals during the Second World War. A common strategy often used by those responsible for such atrocities was that of 'dehumanization' or treating fellow beings as non-persons. This was the ploy used by the Nazis persecuting the Jews, and similar strategies were alleged to have been used by US soldiers describing 'the enemy' in Vietnam and by other war-time personnel (Ife, 2012). It has been suggested that at some level, relating to people as sub-human can make committing acts of atrocity easier and more acceptable (Ife, 2012).

Sadly, there are similarities between such strategies and how some individuals living with dementia were traditionally related to, where the biomedicalization of dementia and its clinical/technical focus often meant that the person was identified as *being the disease* rather than *having the disease* (McLean, 2007), when much less was known about the salience of the social, psychological, economic and cultural aspects of dementia (Bond, 2001), when the person was stripped of personhood (Brock, 1988) and virtually all behaviour and performance was, because of 'dementia', pathologized (Sabat, 2014) and responded to using a medical value base.

Referring to care practices that adopted this technical, clinical and biomedical approach, Kitwood coined the term the *old culture of care* (Kitwood, 1995). In this old culture, dementias were characterised as '... devastating diseases of the central nervous system, in which personality and identity are progressively destroyed' (Kitwood, 1997a, p 136). In this old culture, service providers were often encouraged to eschew their emotions or, in Kitwood's own words, 'in the process of care the key thing is to set aside our own concerns, feelings, vulnerabilities etc, and get on with the job in a sensible, effective way' (Kitwood, 1997a, p 136), and to concentrate on the instrumental tasks of caring. This depersonalization, distancing or abandoning of human emotions was, according to Kitwood and Bredin (1992), done to avoid painful insights, and created what Kitwood (1997a) described as 'us/them' barriers. Here, again, Kitwood left his analysis incomplete, since he failed to argue that the process of depersonalization may have inadvertently legitimated and promoted dehumanizing practices or, as stated by Kontos and Naglie (2007, p 551), the idea that '... there is no affront to human dignity in treating those ... cognitively impaired as though they are unable to experience humiliation.'

Over the last two decades and across the world, several writers (Post, 2000; Innes et al, 2004; Innes, 2009; O'Connor and Purves, 2009; Bartlett and O'Connor, 2010) along with Kitwood, (1990, 1993a, b, 1995, 1997a, b) have challenged the misguided beliefs and inhumane assumptions held by those who believed that dementia stripped people of their personhood, and a significant body of literature now exists that points to the humanity and personhood (Post, 2000; Nuffield Council on Bioethics, 2009; Hughes, 2011, 2014; Flynn and Arstein-Kerslake, 2014), levels of awareness (Clare et al, 2005, 2014) and selfhood (Sabat, 2005) the individual living with dementia continues to have. As noted by Innes (2009), the field of dementia studies constitutes part of a rapidly evolving body of knowledge. According to her, recognition needs to be given to the rights of people living with dementia and to an agenda that embraces humanitarian values such as social inclusion, social justice and citizenship.

Dementia as a health condition

Apart from being a human rights issue, dementia is also a health condition, and globally, over the years, a normative commitment to the right to health (as opposed to a right to being healthy) has been embedded in many human rights treaties (Tobin, 2012). This right to health was first enshrined in the WHO's *Constitution*, which states that everyone has the right to the highest attainable standard of health (WHO, 1946). Later it was recognized in Article 25(1), of the UDHR (UN, 1948). In international law, the right to health has been enshrined in various international human rights treaties (Tobin, 2012).

So far, this chapter has argued that human rights are equal rights that all of us possess because we are human. A rights-based perspective means dismantling the barriers to social participation and to a meaningful life the individual may encounter, and inspiring confidence and hope in the person to self-advocate (Ife, 2012). Hughes (2010) suggests it means asking pertinent questions about people's fundamental rights. Examples might include: how do certain actions such as attaching electronic devices (wrist or ankle bands) on the individual's body or ignoring a request from a vulnerable individual for immediate assistance impact on the person's human rights? A rights-based approach also includes a structural analysis, linking the personal to the political, and recognizing the need to understand problems in their social, historical and political contexts. A rights-based approach is motivated by ethical concerns for social justice, fairness and equality. It is a discourse of hope (Degener, 2014), concentrating on what is wrong but also promoting a vision of what is right. A human rights perspective is about power relations (McGettrick, 2014), and about fostering and promoting human rights to create a fairer, more equitable, world.

Critical perspectives

How dementia is defined and conceptualized and how we approach dementia, greatly influences what are considered legitimate needs (Downs et al, 2006; Innes et al, 2012). These starting points from around which we frame dementia also impact on policy, practice and research (Innes et al, 2012). The content of this book has been influenced by a number of different critical perspectives, and the section that follows now briefly outlines these perspectives, and indicates how each has helped inform the chapters.

Disability studies

Disability studies, which is sometimes considered transdisciplinary, came to the fore in the 1990s and emerged in similar ways to feminist and black studies. Over the years, disability studies have made significant in-roads into disciplines that traditionally marginalized those experiencing a disability, such as medical sociology, philosophy and psychology. A core argument marshalled by the early disability studies writers is that it is not *impairment* that causes *disability*, but rather, that disability is caused by the barriers (social, attitudinal and environmental) non-disabled people erect in society that limit people's active participation. Whilst the early disability writers made a very clear distinction between 'impairment' and 'disability', second-wave writers integrated people's experiences of both impairments and disability, and acknowledged the need to consider both (Shakespeare, 2014).

Collectively, some people with disabilities have highlighted the material conditions of exclusion that have served to disadvantage them (Oliver, 1990) whilst simultaneously developing responses (individual and political) to normalizing disability in society. Today, the field of disability studies continues to develop, in ways inclusive of people experiencing impairments and disability, and those committed to disability studies regard their subject matter as social, political and cultural (Goodley, 2011; WHO and The World Bank, 2011; García Iriarte et al, 2016). Disability studies is also a broad field and contains some notable controversies including the fact that it is dominated by white, middle to upper class, educated people (Albrecht et al, 2001), and as a cognate discipline, disability studies are ageist (Gilliard et al, 2005; Jönson and Larsson, 2009). The mantra of disability activists percolating through to the dementia community (Bryden, 2015) has been 'nothing about us without us' (Charlton, 1998). Although the field of disability studies has helped inform dementia studies, the potential for richer dialogue and collaboration to arise between both cognate disciplines is huge. This issue is explored in more depth in Chapter Two of this book.

Social constructionism

Social constructionism, a viewpoint that adopts a relativist rather than positivist position, has also influenced the writing of this book. Proponents of social constructionism contend that we construct the world we live in, in our social relationships with others – 'the realities we live in are outcomes of the conversations in which we are engaged' (Gergen, 2009, p 4). Social constructionism places an emphasis on language and how it is used to construct reality (Andrews, 2012). It challenges us to re-consider virtually everything we have learned about the world and ourselves (Gergen, 2009) and to consider what the world means to us. Almost all efforts of social constructionists are concerned with social change (Gergen, 2009). The social constructionist perspective, it is argued, fits well with the diversity and complexity of the experiences of living with dementia (Corner and Bond, 2004; Bartlett and O'Connor, 2010). Drawing on this critical perspective, one of the aims of this book is to shed light on how people living with dementia and their family members make sense of their own worlds. This is done by wherever possible drawing on their own rich narratives.

Critical social gerontology

Critical social gerontology also offers a social science framework for bringing together the thoughts and ideas articulated in this work. Critical social gerontology that examines power relations and structural inequalities in society that foster current understandings of ageing (Estes et al, 2003) can also be effectively applied to a critical analysis of dementia. Understanding dementia from a critical, gerontological perspective requires recognition of how older people's experiences are shaped by wider social and political forces, including public attitudes to dementia, stigma and the broader social forces impacting on the individual, including resources allocated to dementia (Innes and Manthorpe, 2013). A critical, gerontological perspective acknowledges that dementia must be examined from a life course perspective, and must include the experiences of diverse groups (Hulko, 2009), including those from different educational and ethnic backgrounds.

Human rights

Finally, a human rights perspective has also informed the approach adopted in this book. This perspective is about empowering the individual to be aware of and claim their rights (SHRC, 2010). It is about training practitioners in human rights principles, and encouraging them to use a rights-based framework in their daily work (Kelly and Innes, 2012). It is also about ensuring that the standards and principles of human rights are incorporated into policy-making (SHRC, 2010). Awareness of human rights and cross-checking policies and programmes to ensure they are compliant with human rights principles and legislation is essential to protecting the interests and dignity of people living with dementia (Mental Health Foundation, 2015; WHO, 2016). Likewise, adopting a human rights-based approach in practice provides a useful framework to enable health service professionals and other dementia care staff to reflect on their practices and address inequities in service provision (Kelly and Innes, 2012).

Bringing together these perspectives, this book attempts to:

- contextualize dementia as a human rights issue with a broad focus on social justice, equality, non-discrimination, autonomy, dignity, social inclusion, participation and solidarity;
- frame dementia as a disability, drawing on both the social model of disability (Oliver, 1990, 1996) and the biopsychosocial model of disability and health (WHO, 2001);
- take cognizance of the principles, objectives and several Articles set out in the CRPD, and operationalize these in order to enhance practice and inform policy;
- create an awareness of how rights-based initiatives embodying human rights principles can generate change in dementia policy and can improve quality of life and quality of care;
- consider the extent to which public policy on dementia takes cognizance of human rights issues;
- provide the analytical tools to enable health service professionals and care workers to interrogate practice and improve quality of care;
- provide the tools for policy-makers to ensure that public policy on dementia is rights-based;
- generate insights into rights-based initiatives in dementia across the world (examples are drawn from the DAI and the *Charter of rights for people with dementia and their carers in Scotland*).

Structure of the book

This book is divided into two parts. Part One provides the conceptual framework and contains three chapters. This chapter has introduced the reader to the broad and complex topic of human rights and dementia, which I have attempted to simplify. I have defined what human rights are, described how human rights are typically classified, explained the origins of the *Universal Declaration of Human Rights* (UN, 1948), and shown how it differs from the *European Convention on Human Rights*. I have argued that dementia is a human rights issue since many people who have the syndrome experience inequality, marginalization, discrimination, social exclusion and at the extreme, social oppression. I have also discussed the key differences between the terms 'needs' and 'rights', and in so doing have briefly critiqued Kitwood's works. The rationale behind writing this book, along with its broad aims and objectives and the critical perspectives drawn on to inform my theorizing, have also been introduced.

Chapter Two draws on the extant literature to deconstruct dementia from a disability perspective. It demonstrates that whilst dementia has conventionally been framed in biomedical terms, conceptualizing it as a disability forces us to look beyond the individual and the disease, to consider the way in which society, through attitudinal, environmental and social barriers, can at times oppress the individual. A central theme underpinning this chapter is how dementia has remained under-represented in disability studies, and whilst the two cognate disciplines (dementia studies and disability studies) are beginning to enter into dialogue with each other, there is a need for much stronger collaboration. In the final part of the chapter reasons are put forward as to why the individual living with dementia falls within the CRPD description of a person with a disability, and therefore has full entitlement to each of the human rights the Convention enshrines. Demonstrating why dementia qualifies as a disability in line with the CRPD is important, given how this book explores the rights of people living with dementia to claim entitlements set out in the CRPD.

Chapter Three focuses on the CRPD, and shows that as an instrument of social change, it provides a legitimate springboard for the reframing of dementia as a disability and as a human rights issue, and for the emergence of reform in dementia policy and practice. The Articles selected for later critical review in this book are identified in this chapter. Some recommendations are forwarded about how Articles in the CRPD could be re-worked to make them more inclusive of the individual living with dementia. The chapter concludes with a brief discussion of some recent political developments that reflect the gradual emergence of a rights–based movement occurring in dementia policy and practice.

In Part Two which interrogates dementia policy and practice, Chapter Four expands public discourse on dementia as a social justice issue by exploring a number of rights most of us take for granted that are often restricted for those living with dementia. In particular, the chapter addresses the individual's right to be treated equally before the law, the right to a timely diagnosis, its ethical disclosure, the right to rehabilitation based on a multidisciplinary assessment, and to live well with dementia in the community with personal supports. The chapter argues that in England, Ireland and across several European countries, there is a lack of commitment in government policy to providing access to social care that would otherwise enable people to exercise their social rights to live in the community.

Chapter Five reports on some of the basic human rights people living in long-term residential care should be afforded but are sometimes denied. These include the right to be protected from cruel, inhuman or degrading treatment or punishment, the right to privacy, to access outdoor areas and to participate in cultural life, recreational and leisure activities. The chapter argues that much of the excess disability experienced by people living with dementia in long-term care settings arises as a result of social, economic and environmental barriers. Some of these barriers may be easily eliminated but others will need considerable resources and a change in the culture of care. The chapter demonstrates how the biomedical model for understanding and responding to dementia still prevails in many long-term care settings where the dominant focus continues to be on clinical management, drug treatments and policies of restriction and control.

Chapter Six explores the implications of a human rights-based approach for dementia policy and practice. Revisiting the issues discussed in earlier chapters I argue that much of the debate about the human rights of people with dementia focuses on the protection of negative rights, including the right to respect, autonomy, dignity and non-discrimination, but not on positive economic and social rights, including the right to participate in one's local community and remain socially engaged. Findings from a recent survey conducted with healthcare professionals and care staff, investigating their attitudes to human rights issues, are presented. It is shown how a rights-based discourse has, by and large, failed to penetrate current iterations of most national dementia strategies. The importance of ensuring that practitioners undergo rights-based training is emphasised in this chapter, and some synergies are drawn between elements of person-centred care and rights-based principles.

Chapter Seven investigates the concepts of autonomy and capacity, particularly as they relate to Article 12 of the CRPD and the more recent General Comment on Article 12. The chapter provides definitions of legal and mental capacity, and argues that functional tests of mental capacity that lead to the denial of legal capacity violate this Article. Two examples of law reform on legal capacity from Ireland and Canada are discussed and reference is made to the proposed new UN Convention on the Rights of Older People.

Chapter Eight summarizes the key themes emerging from each of the preceding chapters, and brings them together in a discussion centring on two broad topics – 'grounds for hope' and 'a life of quality and equality'. In this chapter I argue that there are grounds to be optimistic for a future world where people diagnosed with dementia and those who support them can live well and enjoy a good quality of life. The research, practice and policy implications emerging from discussions in this book are also highlighted in this chapter, as is the salience of the new global action plan on dementia (WHO, 2016). An appeal is made for more resources to be allocated to dementia.

A brief word on terminology

It is well known that the language we use informs and reflects our understanding of the world in which we live (Barnes and Mercer, 2010) and the everyday language used to describe a person living with dementia can significantly influence perceptions and attitudes to dementia (George, 2010), and can impact on the individual (Swaffer, 2014). Throughout this book, and as far as possible, I follow the terminology and non-stigmatizing, inclusive language recommended by Alzheimer's Australia (2014). Consequently I avoid using words like 'patient', 'sufferer' or 'demented person' (except when italicized and as quoted by others), and refer to the individual as a 'person living with dementia', very occasionally abbreviating these words to 'they'. However, I am conscious that no two people with dementia are the same, and that there is a huge diversity amongst individuals. Accordingly, in my use of the word 'they', I do not lose sight of the individual, whose only attribute not shared with the rest of us without dementia is a diagnosis of dementia. Similarly I steer clear of using words like 'family caregiver', except where the concept was the main focus of earlier studies, since I believe that this places the individual in a subordinate position. Instead I use the term 'family member'. Throughout the book I use the term 'behaviours that challenge' or, with reference to the clinical contexts, the expression 'behavioural and psychological symptoms of dementia'. What is important here is not political correctness, but rather choosing respectful, empowering language that focuses on abilities and that will help to challenge some of the myths about dementia still held in some societies today (Cahill et al, 2015b).

Summary of key points

- Human rights are basic rights that everyone is entitled to – they are about how the state and others treat the individual.
- Human rights can be classified as civil, political, economic, social and cultural.
- Civil and political rights are commonly known as *negative rights*, which means that they require protection against abuse, whilst economic, social and cultural rights are commonly known as *positive rights*, which means they place a claim on others for positive assistance.
- The atrocities and violations that occurred during the Second World War led to the need to create a more peaceful world and to the launch of the *Universal Declaration of Human Rights* (UN, 1948).
- The *Universal Declaration of Human Rights* was the first global, explicit commitment to the fact that human rights are an essential entitlement of all human beings.
- Dementia is a human rights issue since the individual diagnosed is at heightened risk of experiencing inequalities, injustices, marginalization and discrimination.
- Dementia is also a health condition, and rights to health were first enshrined in the WHO's (1946) *Constitution*, which states that everyone has the right to the highest attainable standard of health. This right to health was later recognized in the *Universal Declaration of Human Rights*.
- Conceptually, human rights are different from human needs.
- Kitwood's theorizing of dementia focused specifically on the human needs as opposed to the human rights of the individual.
- A rights-based approach to policy and practice provides a strong moral framework for addressing social and political change.

TWO

Dementia as a disability

Introduction

In Chapter One, the topic of human rights and dementia was introduced, and it was shown that dementia is a human rights issue since the individual diagnosed can experience injustice, inequality and marginalization. As I argue in later chapters, once diagnosed a person may encounter discrimination, segregation and social exclusion (Cantley and Bowes, 2004), their autonomy can be compromised (Boyle, 2008), and opportunities to exercise choice and control in decisions directly relevant to their lives may be denied (Nuffield Council on Bioethics, 2009; Hughes, 2011). The individual may also be subjected to other injustices (Post, 2000; Bartlett, 2016), including prejudicial and stereotypical attitudes (Bartlett and O'Connor, 2010; Dupuis et al, 2016) and to unhelpful, and at times, harmful, interventions (Banerjee, 2009).

Apart from being a human rights issue, dementia can also be framed as a disability (Kitwood, 1993a, 1997a; Bartlett, 2000; Beattie et al, 2005; Gilliard et al, 2005; Marshall, 2005; Dorenlot, 2005; Thomas and Milligan, 2015; Mental Health Foundation, 2015; Hare, 2016; Shakespeare et al, 2017), although the inclusion of dementia in disability studies and conversely, the integration of the concepts and tools generated by disability scholars into dementia studies, has been slow to evolve (Shakespeare et al, 2017). Indeed, at a recent conference (Mittler, 2016b), an academic, who has self-identified as having both dementia and a disability, commented on this same disconnect when he said: "Dementia and disability seem like planets spinning on different axes, their inhabitants aware of each other's existence but apparently unable to communicate. There is a perception in the disability world that dementia is solely a health responsibility. People with dementia do not necessarily think of themselves as disabled." This disconnection reflects missed opportunities since contextualizing dementia as a disability can, as I will argue in this chapter, yield benefit.

This chapter draws on the extant literature, especially critical writings from disability studies, to re-examine dementia from a disability perspective, and to demonstrate the unique challenges that confront self-advocates who have dementia, when campaigning for their rights. Using tools derived from disability studies, a secondary aim of the chapter is to build on different models of disability to provide a compelling argument as to why dementia should be framed as a disability, and to outline the opportunities available to the dementia community by placing dementia under a disability lens. A central theme threading through the chapter is that dementia has consistently remained under-represented in disability studies (Bartlett, 2014; Shakespeare et al, 2017).

Conceptualizing dementia as a disability is not entirely new (see also for example Sabat, 1994; Marshall, 1998, 2001; Blackman et al, 2003; Manthorpe et al, 2003; Bartlett, 2014). However, the task here is to extend the debate by exploring in greater depth the opportunities to be gained from such conceptualizations and in so doing, build on and critique earlier works. Given how the CRPD is the prism through which dementia policy and practice is examined in this book, a later part of this chapter focuses on demonstrating that people living with dementia fall within the CRPD description of disability and therefore have full rights to the provisions set out in the Convention. At the outset it should be emphasised that by framing dementia as a disability, it is not intended to downplay the importance of regarding it as a health issue (Crowther, 2015) and medical problem. All perspectives are said to 'offer insights in exchange for some limitation in approach' (Silverman, 1970, p 44).

Language is a powerful tool, and its use can be an 'important indicator of views and stereotypes in both disability studies and in dementia care' (Gilliard et al, 2005, p 577). Words and phrases can be used to sustain, reinforce or challenge stereotypes (Alzheimer's Australia, 2014). At the end of this chapter, therefore, a critique of the language used in dominant discourse on dementia is undertaken, and an appeal is made for balanced 'messaging'. But first, to a critical review of the key debates on contemporary definitions of disability, and to a discussion of their relevance to the field of dementia studies. In recasting dementia as a disability, three different models are critiqued here, namely, the (i) biomedical, (ii) social and (iii) biopsychosocial. It is shown that the application of these particular models to interrogate dementia allows for a richer understanding of dementia as a disability, and enables us identify useful practice and research tools.

Defining disability

Approximately 1 billion people around the world have a disability, a figure representing 15 per cent of the world's population (WHO and The World Bank, 2011). Even though dementia rarely features within official reports on disability, the figure of 1 billion is said to include people living with dementia (Marianne Schulz, personal communication, 2016). In Europe, some 45 per cent of people with a disability are aged 65 and over (ENNHRI, 2016). Given the magnitude of disability therefore, and the significant gains made by a burgeoning disability rights movement, disability remains a complex, contentious, multi-dimensional and dynamic construct (WHO and The World Bank, 2011), and depending on what purpose is intended (Altman, 2001; García Iriarte, 2016), multiple definitions of disability exist. Disability studies – a branch of knowledge that examines the *meaning,* nature and consequences of *'disability'* as a social construct – has expanded rapidly since the 1990s when it first emerged as an academic discipline. Today a lot more is known about the meaning and experience of disability than in the past, when the medical profession held supremacy, the biomedical model remained dominant (Oliver, 1989), and when people with a 'handicap'[1] were generally looked upon as 'victims of a tragic happening' (Oliver, 1990, p 2), sometimes labelled as 'retarded', pitied and patronised (Shakespeare, 2006; Goodley and Runswick-Cole, 2011).

Models of disability

Broadly speaking models are representations of concepts that help us understand and can assist in decision-making. Models can help organize conceptual elements and can be used to translate ideas into practice (Oliver, 2004). Many different models of disability have been developed both within and outside the field of disability studies (Degener, 2014; see also García Iriarte, 2016, for a comprehensive overview and critique of disability models).

The biomedical model

The biomedical model considers '… disability as an impairment that needs to be treated, cured, fixed or at least rehabilitated' (Degener, 2014, p 3). It is a model underpinned by a personal tragedy theory of disability (Oliver, 1989), with loss being the chosen metaphor through which all behaviour is understood. Disability is regarded as a medical problem, a deviation from 'normal' health status (Degener, 2014), and disability is seen to reside in the individual because of an impairment (Goodley, 2011). 'Patients' are expected to passively use services offered by trained healthcare professionals, and their disability 'needs to be cured by medical and rehabilitation professionals' (García Iriarte, 2016, p 14).

Over the years the biomedical model has been heavily critiqued (Oliver, 1990; Degener, 2014; Shakespeare, 2014) for its reductionism and bias, for placing undue emphasis on pathology and on clinical diagnosis (Oliver, 1990), for seeing people exclusively through their disability, and for viewing all difficulties as being amenable to treatments (Brisenden, 1986). Despite these limitations and the only partial insights it affords, the biomedical model continues to be the most dominant paradigm used for resource allocation in disability services and, indeed, in more affluent countries, the biomedical model is highly influential in determining welfare benefits (Oliver, 1990; García Iriarte, 2016).

First emerging in the US and UK during the late 1960s and 1970s, and probably influenced by the rise in social movements including gay and lesbian, working-class and black civil rights, a disability movement gradually began to gain traction across the world. In the UK, disability activists organized themselves around local issues such as their exclusion from community living (Oliver, 1983; Barnes, 1991). Local issues then escalated to national concerns, which, in turn, led to the establishment of disabled people's organizations (Bartlett, 2000). These disability activists were instrumental in questioning the meaning of 'disability' and the ideas and practices they believed oppressed people with disabilities (Oliver, 1990).

The core argument marshalled by these activists was that 'disability' was socially constructed (Goodley, 2011) – people with disabilities were not disadvantaged because of their 'impairments', but rather because of the negative responses and barriers society erected against them (Thomas and Milligan, 2015). They coined the term 'disablism' to mean 'the social imposition of avoidable restrictions on the life activities, aspirations and psycho-emotional wellbeing of people categorized as "impaired" by those deemed "normal"' (Thomas, 2010, p 37). In the UK the early disability writers campaigned for greater autonomy and control in residential institutions, for new living options, and for an adequate disability income (Barnes and Mercer, 2010), and pointed to the multiple types of oppression including racism, ageism and sexism people with disabilities experience (Gilson and Depoy, 2000).

The social model

Building on the earlier work (1976) of the Union of Physically Impaired Against Segregation (UPIAS), in 1983, Oliver, a UK-based physically disabled academic, coined the term the 'social model of disability'. Stated simply, this model identifies society rather than the individual as the core source of disability, and proponents of this model claim that solutions to disability are found not in curing the 'impairment' (a biological explanation), but by challenging discrimination and social disadvantage (a socio-political explanation). These early disability writers carefully differentiated between the concepts of 'impairment' and 'disability', concerned that any attention focused on impairment would detract attention from the oppression caused to people with disabilities by society (Oliver, 1996). Interestingly, 'impairments' were regarded by them as physical and not mental or cognitive (UPIAS, 1976). In fact, the invisibility of cognitive impairment and mental health issues in the original conceptualization of the social model of disability is well illustrated in *Fundamental principles of disability* (UPIAS, 1976), an authoritative document that provided the framework for the social model. In this document, the definition of impairment and disability was:

> Thus we define *impairment* as lacking part of or all of a limb, or having a defective limb organ or mechanism of the body; and *disability* as the disadvantage or restriction of activity caused by a contemporary social organization which takes no or little account of people who have physical impairments and thus excludes them from participation in the mainstream of social activities. *Physical disability* is therefore a particular form of social oppression. (UPIAS, 1976, p 14; emphasis added)

The social model has been critiqued for its almost exclusive focus on the body rather than the mind as the main source of impairment, for its concern with structure and the built environment to the detriment of agency and practice, and for its exclusion of people with dementia from analysis, since their impairments are seen as cognitive and not physical (Owens, 2015). Goodley (2001) argues that in relegating 'impairments' to biological deficits, people with a cognitive impairment feel discriminated against. Deal (2003) asserts that there is a hierarchy of impairments amongst people with disabilities, and the individual with dementia is located at the bottom of this hierarchy. Others (see, for example, Gilliard et al, 2005) contend that the neglect of older people, including those with dementia, in disability studies is essentially ageist. Yet despite its numerous limitations, the social model is a powerful tool that can be used in advocacy campaigns. In fact, it is said to have much potential for people living with dementia (Dornelot, 2005; Mental Health Foundation, 2015; Hare, 2016), and for those keen to analyse oppressive and discriminatory structures in society (Degener, 2014).

The biopsychosocial model

Since the late 1990s, a variation of the social model began to emerge, and a more holistic approach to conceptualizing disability evolved amongst 'second-wave' writers (Deal, 2003). This more holistic approach reflecting the biopsychosocial model is best exemplified in the International Classification of Functioning, Disability and Health (ICF) proposed by WHO (2001). The ICF has two parts: the first deals with functioning and disability while the second relates to contextual factors. In the first part, three interconnected areas of functionality are identified, namely: (i) impairments, defined by WHO (2001, p 12) as 'problems in body function such as a significant deviation or loss'; (ii) activity limitations, defined by WHO (2001, p 12) as 'difficulties an individual may have in executing activities' and; (iii) participation restrictions, defined by WHO (2001, p 12) as 'problems an individual may experience in involvement in life situations'. According to the first part of this model (see Figure 2.1) difficulties arising in any one, two or in all three of these areas constitute a disability (WHO and The World Bank, 2011).

Figure 2.1: Disability arising due to difficulties relating to impairments or activity limitations or participation restrictions or all three

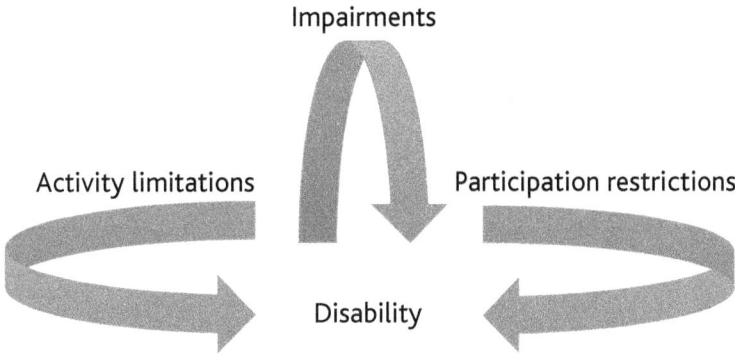

Impairments

Activity limitations

Participation restrictions

Disability

Source: Figure 2.1 developed based on information from WHO (2001) and from WHO and the World Bank Report, (2011)
Note: Figure 2.1 and Figure 2.2 should be read in combination

Part two of the model considers functioning and disability as a 'dynamic interaction between health conditions and contextual factors both environmental and personal factors' (WHO and The World Bank, 2011, p 4). Environmental factors are extrinsic to the individual and refer to 'the physical, social, and attitudinal environment in which people live and conduct their lives' (WHO, 2001, p 12). Personal factors are intrinsic to the individual and include, 'gender, race, age, other health conditions fitness, lifestyle, habits, upbringing, …' (WHO, 2001, p 23). These personal factors may impede or facilitate functioning and will influence how a disability is experienced and the extent to which a person can or cannot fully participate in society.

Figure 2.2: Disability arising from the interaction of health conditions and contextual factors

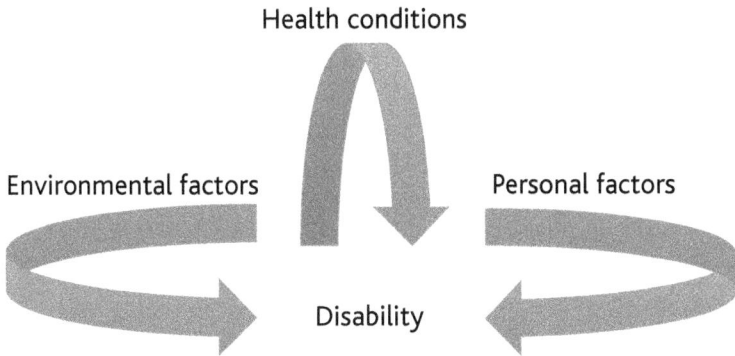

Health conditions

Environmental factors

Personal factors

Disability

Source: Figure 2.2 developed based on information from WHO (2001) and from WHO and the World Bank Report, (2011)

The biopsychosocial model as reflected in the ICF is universal insofar as it applies to all human functioning, and it places equal emphasis on the health condition and the role contextual factors play in determining health and wellbeing. Importantly, the biopsychosocial model, as exemplified in the ICF (WHO, 2001), differentiates between a person's capacity to perform actions and the actual performance, showing how performance can be improved by adjusting/manipulating the environment (WHO and The World Bank, 2011). Over the years the biopsychosocial model has been successfully applied in several research studies on Alzheimer's disease and dementia (see, for example, Arthanat et al, 2004; Hagen et al, 2004; Muò et al, 2005; Pierce et al, 2015; Revolta et al, 2016).

Models of dementia

The biomedical model

As mentioned, different models used to enhance our understanding of disability have also been applied to reframe dementia. There are parallels between how disability has been conceptualized traditionally and how dementia has been recast over the last three decades, since, until recently, the biomedical model, focusing on neuropathological explanations, has dominated our thinking on dementia (Innes, 2009; O'Shea and Carney, 2016), and dementia has almost exclusively been seen through a diseased brain lens (Blessed et al, 1968; Finnema et al, 2000). This lens assumes the existence of a straightforward, causal relationship between neuropathology and dementia (Bond, 1992). By focusing on the neuropathology and on the diseased and atrophied brain and not on the person, the biomedical model is said to squeeze out the individual (Stokes and Goudie, 2002). It is a lens that regards dementia as a progressive neuro-degenerative brain disorder, and hones in on the underlying pathology causing the disease and on treatments (Taft et al, 1997). As a cognitive disorder, dementia is characterized by intellectual deterioration and, at later stages, by the erosion of mental and physical function (NICE/SCIE, 2007). This biomedical framing of dementia is said to focus principally on deficits, and virtually ignores intact, retained abilities (Sabat, 2011). It is regarded by some as overly scientific and does not consider the patient to be an active partner in the treatment process (Vogt et al, 2014).

Whilst many dementias lack biomarkers (Gabel et al, 2010), and there are still no effective disease-modifying treatments available (Winblad et al, 2016), nonetheless, the biomedical model of dementia, with its focus on pathology, aetiology, pharmacology and prognosis (Bond et al, 2002), continues to prevail, and it is said that, 'dementia still remains trapped within the dominant medical discourse' (Shakespeare et al, 2017, p 4). Today, most research funding dedicated to dementia results from how the illness has been conceptualized and responded to medically, clinically and pharmacologically (Wu et al, 2015; Batsch, 2016) and not socially, psychologically or politically (Innes, 2009). Like disability, the personal tragedy discourse for dementia (Dupuis et al, 2016) has also been used to explain the effect dementia has on the individual and on family members. Despite its shortcomings, the biomedical model remains critical to our understanding of dementia as it helps to ensure that the individual receives a diagnosis and has access to relevant drug treatments that may, in the short term, slow down cognitive decline and alleviate functional and behavioural symptoms (O'Shea and Carney, 2016).

The social model

Similar to how disability activists had, during the 1960s and 1970s, challenged the biomedical model of disability, in the 1980s and early 1990s, several writers, principally sociologists, and as cited by Innes (2009) (see, for example, Gubrium, 1986; Lyman, 1989; Bond, 1992), began questioning the biomedical model of dementia. It was argued that the disease model was a social construction developed to address 'society's prevailing concern for order and control' (Innes, 2009, p 8). This type of theorizing acted as a catalyst for the development of the social model of dementia, an approach that draws on the social model of disability (Bond, 2001) and focuses on the attitudinal and structural barriers society erects, which oppress people and restrict their participation in society (Thomas and Milligan, 2015). The social model recognizes that dementia is both a disability as well as a medical condition for which there is no cure (O'Shea and Carney, 2016). It emphasizes the way in which the individual and family members interpret their experiences of living with dementia, the meaning their situation has for them and the efforts they make to participate as social citizens in society (Bond, 2001). In this way the individual's response to the dementia is central to the social model (Bond, 2001).

Dementia is considered within a life course perspective, and is only one of a number of ways in which an individual's personal and social capacities may change (NICE/SCIE, 2007). Proponents of the social model assert that people diagnosed have rights: they should be treated equally, and seen as 'a legitimate part of mainstream society, living in communities as equal citizens with their value recognized and respected' (Mental Health Foundation, 2015, p 21). Proponents of the social model still hold out hope for a medical cure (Mental Health Foundation, 2015), but do not see pharmacological treatment as the sole solution. Reframing dementia in social terms has the potential to improve the life of the individual, similar to what the social model of disability has achieved for people with disabilities (O'Shea and Carney, 2016).

The biopsychosocial model

In more recent years, the influences of the biomedical model and social model have been advanced and augmented by the insightful contributions made by a number of social and clinical scientists whose thinking and framing of dementia has more than likely been influenced by the ICF (WHO, 2001). These writers and researchers (see, for example, Hughes, 2011, 2014; Sabat, 2011; Mishra and Barratt, 2016; Spector et al, 2016; Revolta et al, 2016; Clare, 2017) adopt a broader framework by subscribing to a biopsychosocial model. This model focuses on the totality of the individual, and highlights what a person can experience and achieve irrespective of the severity of the dementia (Sabat, 2011). It takes a whole-person approach to understanding dementia, and considers the wide range of factors including biological, psychological, social, economic and environmental, likely to impact on the individual's subjective experience (O'Shea and Carney, 2016).

Although not explicitly spelt out at the time, Kitwood's (1993b) framing of dementia, in which he argued that dementia should first be seen as a disability reflects this biopsychosocial approach, since, for Kitwood, senile dementia (SD) occurred as a result of the complex interaction between one's personality, (P) biography, (B) health (H), neurological impairment (NI) and social psychology (SP) and Kitwood then used the equation 'SD=P+B+H+NI +SP' (Kitwood, 1993a, p 541) to reflect this. Although Kitwood referred to the biomedical model as old fashioned and problematic, he never negated its value, but rather questioned why dementia was always framed only as an organic mental disorder (Kitwood, 1997a), and why society was so preoccupied with explaining 'the pathological processes and then find[ing] ways of arresting or prevent[ing] them' (Kitwood, 1997a, p 1).

Likewise, Marshall (1998, 2001, 2005) who, like Kitwood (1993b, 1997a), framed dementia as a disability (Marshall, 1994) characterised by multiple impairments, and who created an inclusive model of dementia, 'selecting the most helpful elements from many views'

(Gilliard et al, 2005, p 575), also subscribes to the biopsychosocial model. Similarly Sabat's earlier conceptualizations of dementia (1994), where he discussed the 'excess disability' meaning the additional disability that people often experience because of unsupportive and unsympathetic interactions (Sabat, 1994), was also underpinned by a broader biopsychosocial framework. For Sabat, excess disability was '[the] discrepancy that exists when a person's functional incapacity is greater than that warranted by the actual impairment' (Sabat, 1994, p 158), and building on both his and his colleagues' earlier exploration of selfhood in dementia (Sabat and Harré, 1992), Sabat (1994) used a case study to show the type of excess disability (in this case, reduced self-esteem) beyond the neuropathological problem a person can experience due to adverse contextual (environmental and personal) factors.

A critique of Kitwood

Despite successfully reframing dementia as a disability and their enormous contributions to the field of dementia studies, it could be argued that neither Kitwood, Sabat nor Marshall's analysis took advantage of the language and tools developed and adopted by disability scholars and disability rights activists over the years. None, for example, called for political or legislative change to promote the autonomy and wellbeing of people living with dementia and to improve their quality of life. Kitwood and Sabat's theorizing drew heavily on case studies and on clinical and social psychology (personhood, selfhood, interpersonal relations), and not on disability studies (disabilism, oppression, discrimination). Marshall's analysis drew on a public health paradigm of dementia and not on critical social gerontology (socio-political structures, social systems and power relations in society) or on disability studies. In addition, although successfully recasting dementia as a disability and pointing to how the individual could be supported and empowered, depending on the nature and quality of social interactions, none exhorted people living with dementia to act as self-advocates and become politically active.

Kitwood's analysis was reductionist. He contended that personhood (see Chapter One for a definition) could be eroded by the harmful actions (often unintentional) of carers, and not by the inertness and inactivity of political systems and by governments' failure to prioritise and set realistic budgets to provide the resources needed for good dementia support and care. Kitwood (1993a, pp 542-3) referred to concepts of, 'treachery, disempowerment, infantilization, condemnation, intimidation, stigmatization, outpacing, invalidation, banishment and objectification' as elements of 'malignant social psychology' (how the environment can make things worse for the person), and not to discrimination, marginalization, social exclusion and social inequality. Whilst his analysis was revolutionary and provided fresh insights, it was limited since it focused on the care environment and on practice issues, solutions to which could be found in staff training and in organizational/cultural change. In other words, his theorizing honed in more on the *private troubles* of individuals rather than on *public issues* of social systems and institutions (Mills, 1959).

'Ill-being', in Kitwood's view (1997a), resulted from deficiencies in practitioners' skills: the unintentional erosion of personhood caused by the absence of person-centred care and not from ageism, sexism, disablism or the absence of well-developed public policy on dementia. Much dementia care, he contended, was oppressive since carers often lacked the time and skills required to promote personhood and to maintain relationships of trust and respect that might generate a sense of dignity, agency, reassurance and confidence in those they cared for. He asserted that greater attention to the individual's emotional and relational wellbeing would likely counteract some of the adverse behavioural consequences of the neurological impairment (Kitwood, 1997a). Kitwood did not, however, question the meaning of the word *dementia* or coin the term *dementia-ism*, a concept later introduced by Brooker (2004) to reflect a particular type of ageism experienced by people living with dementia.

Success of the disability rights movement: some unique challenges for self advocates diagnosed with dementia

So far an argument has been marshalled about the limitations of regarding dementia exclusively as an organic brain disease and the advantages to be gained in recasting it as a disability. It must be reiterated that conceptualizing dementia as a disability does not negate the salience of recognizing the clinical, biological, neuropathological and neurophysiological aspects of the illness. Specific theoretical perspectives have their merits and demerits: 'many social scientists now recognize that no picture is ever complete, that what is needed is many perspectives, many voices before we can achieve deep understandings of social phenomena and before we can assert that the narrative is complete' (Denzin and Lincoln, 1994, p 580).

However, what I have argued is that over the years, the disability rights movement led by people with disabilities has been extremely successful in challenging the biomedical model and changing the dominant ideology by pointing to the inequities people with disabilities experience because of physical, attitudinal and structural barriers embedded in society. Although a level of social exclusion as reflected in some people continuing to live in congregated settings still exists, broadly speaking, the disability movement has been successful in its lobby for non-discriminatory policies and in developing new legislation to help integrate people with disabilities in society. Some of its most noteworthy achievements include the development of equality and anti-discrimination legislation along with disability legislation, and obtaining improved resources for services and welfare benefits (Thomas and Milligan, 2015). Other important achievements include the elimination of pejorative language (Hughes, 2011) and in so doing, making disability-related language more neutral (Charlton, 2000). Globally, probably the greatest testament to its success lies in the development and adoption of the CRPD, considered to be a landmark treaty in the history of disability rights (García Iriarte, 2016).

Accordingly, in challenging conventional representations of disability, disability activists and disability scholars have transported disability from a status of hopelessness and tragedy to a position of activism and self-determination, where disability has become a societal responsibility (Gilliard et al, 2005). A likely factor explaining its success is that the disability rights movement has been led by and for people with disability whose impairments have been largely visible and who have subscribed to the social model of disability.

In contrast, the dementia movement has, until relatively recently, been led by health service professionals (especially medical doctors such as geriatricians, neurologists, old age psychiatrists, GPs and neuro-psychologists), clinical researchers, pharmaceutical companies and organizations like the ADI and Alzheimer Europe, originally dedicated to preventing dementia, finding a cure, developing treatments and to supporting 'family caregivers'. Historically the movement has not been controlled by individuals experiencing the symptoms: taking the drugs, feeling the side-effects, sometimes being forced against their wishes to enter nursing homes and occasionally being treated like social outcasts and locked indoors. In fact, in the past, had the individual spoken out publicly about such injustices, it is likely their complaints may have been seen as angry outbursts or irrational behaviour (Bartlett, 2000) and possibly 'managed' with drugs.

Self-advocacy is only a relatively new and emerging phenomenon in the dementia space (Glenn Rees, personal communication, 2016), and self-advocates living with dementia face particular challenges. For example the nature of the condition means that only those with a mild to moderate dementia can advocate for themselves (Shakespeare et al, 2017). Much energy is needed to lobby governments, change ideology, challenge deficit models of policy, highlight human rights violations, transform the dominant discourse and represent one's fellow human being whose experiences may be entirely different to that of the self-advocate. No policy or practice should be decided by any representative without the full participation of members of that group most affected, but how exactly can this be achieved for the individual with end-stage dementia in long-term care?

Compared with disability activism, the dementia movement is new, lacks critical mass, the disability is often invisible and many people may be slow to self-identify with a stigmatizing condition. Advocacy organizations representing vulnerable groups will never have the same insights, and the same impact as those lobbying for political change who experience a disability on a day-to-day basis. It takes courage to challenge the biomedical model (O'Sullivan, 2013), and, unlike disability political activists, the individual living with dementia may be ambivalent about challenging healthcare systems when hope still reigns high for a cure (Mental Health Foundation, 2015).

The way forward

I have outlined some of the successes achieved by the disability rights movement and people with disabilities over more recent years. However, in my view their greatest success and indeed legacy to individuals diagnosed with dementia and their families is the CRPD. This is because the rights contained in the CRPD are also directly relevant to the lives of individuals who have dementia and their family members (Mittler, 2015; Rees, 2015; Williamson, 2015; DAI, 2016) *provided the CRPD's definition of 'disability' is inclusive of people living with dementia.* So how is disability defined in the CRPD? Is its definition sufficiently comprehensive to be inclusive of people living with dementia? The next section addresses these two important questions.

Disability and the CRPD

Although much effort was invested into developing a suitable definition of both 'impairment' and 'disability' for the CRPD, no consensus was ever reached (García Iriarte, 2016); indeed, it is noted that at least 50 definitions of disability were forwarded (Schulze, 2010). Accordingly, the CRPD is said to provide a description rather than a definition of disability and disabled people. For a comprehensive understanding of how disability and people with disabilities are described in the CRPD, Schulze (2010) recommends that both the Preamble (description of disability), along with Article 1 (description of disabled people), should be read together. Table 2.1 details both.

Table 2.1: CRPD description of disability and persons with disabilities

CRPD Preamble	Recognizing that disability is an evolving concept and that disability results from the interaction between persons with impairments and attitudinal and environmental barriers that hinders their full and effective participation in society on an equal basis with others
CRPD Article 1	Persons with disabilities include those who have long-term physical, mental, intellectual or sensory impairments, which, in interaction with various barriers, may hinder their full and effective participation in society on an equal basis with others

Source: Schulze (2010)

The influence of the ICF (WHO, 2001) and the biopsychosocial model of disability can be seen in both the CRPD Preamble and in Article 1, where the dynamic dimensions of disability are reflected in its four integrated components, namely (i) impairments, (ii) barriers, (iii) participation and (iv) equality. However, the social model of disability is also evident in the Preamble statement, since the concepts of 'impairment' and 'disability' are clearly differentiated. In terms of Article 1, what is noteworthy in the description of people with a disability is the absence of reference to a *cognitive* impairment. This may be because it is assumed that a 'cognitive impairment' is synonymous with a 'mental impairment' or an 'intellectual impairment'. A simple addition made to Article 1, with the insertion of the word 'cognitive', would mean that in the future people living with dementia would be more explicitly included in the CRPD's description of disability. This is a very minor change I would now recommend.

However, to return to the question of whether people with dementia fit the classification of disability set down in the CRPD, the answer is quite categorically, yes. This is because the Preamble statement emphasises the *impairment* aspects of disability (and we know that dementia causes multiple impairments such as memory, cognitive, including judgement, perception, language, reasoning, and so on). Likewise, the individual diagnosed with dementia is well aligned with Article 1, since it states that people with disabilities include those with long-term physical, mental, intellectual and sensory impairment. Whilst 'dementia is technically a syndrome or set of symptoms, that can be caused by any number of diseases' (Post, 2000, p 4), there is no ambiguity about the fact that in most cases dementia is progressive and irreversible, and causes physical and intellectual impairments (WHO, 2012).

The CRPD is a powerful working tool, which can be used by people living with dementia, their family members and by practitioners and policy-makers working in the field. Its relevance to the lives of the individual and their family members has recently been acknowledged and endorsed by WHO (2016) and by the ADI (Rees, 2017). In later chapters of this book, several of the Articles enshrined in the CRPD will be scrutinized to demonstrate what they actually mean to the everyday life of the individual living with dementia, and to interrogate dementia policy and practice, but first, before doing so, I want to return to the topic of language use in dementia discourse.

Language and dementia

As noted earlier, language is an important tool in public narratives, such as in policy documents, in academic and healthcare literature (Mitchell et al, 2013), and in everyday speech. Words, either written or oral, convey meaning and influence how people perceive themselves (Swaffer, 2014), and how they are perceived by others (Cayton, 2006). The media and the language it uses informs people's attitudes, beliefs and assumptions on a wide variety of topics, and the choice of words and phrases used in media communications is extremely important in shaping public opinion.

Regrettably, over the years, the media have provided a very biased and often sensationalist account of dementia by using language that depicts it very negatively and by portraying it as a frightening, mysterious, relentless and fatal disease (Hyman, 2008), thereby reinforcing stigma. The language of warfare is also often used where the individual is portrayed as being 'attacked' or 'ravaged' and reduced to a 'non-person' (George, 2010), sometimes even experiencing a 'social death' (Sweeting and Gilhooly, 1997). Curiously this nihilistic and one-sided account of dementia promoted by the media hones in almost exclusively on the middle to end-of-life stages of the condition (van Gorp and Vercruysse, 2012), without providing a more balanced overview. Indeed, it has been noted that the stereotypical portrayal of an individual diagnosed with dementia conveyed by the media is that of a Caucasian, exhibiting a blank stare whilst wandering down a hall or sometimes being hugged by a child (Gray-Vickrey, 2009), or a frail elderly, disorientated person as an escapee from a nursing home. Given this type of sensational imagery, it is not surprising that the public are fearful of dementia (Post, 2000; ADI, 2012). The media fuels this fear by comparing dementia to HIV/AIDS (*Irish Times*, 2015) and by using metaphors such as 'rising tide', 'silent epidemic' (Gove et al, 2015) and words like 'tsunami' (*Irish Examiner*, 2015) to describe prevalence rates.

Swaffer (2014), in a powerful editorial, critically reviews the impact of language on stigma and, like George (2010), contends that governments welcome nihilistic language since it may attract political and budgetary attention and help to garner resources including philanthropic funding. She appeals for balanced messaging and for the use of normal, inclusive and jargon-free language, which is supportive rather than offensive. Honing in on the current global trend to develop dementia-friendly communities, she questions the prudence of expressions such as 'dementia-friendly', suggesting that these words may be divisive and may stigmatize people who have dementia.

Yet, despite such appeals and the increasing attention dementia is attracting in mainstream culture (George, 2010), the 'tragedy meta narrative' (Dupuis et al, 2016) remains dominant in Western society. One consequence of this is that the individual can be made feel very different to others and can experience injustices including the loss of rights (Mitchell et al, 2013). Whilst undoubtedly a person with a cognitive impairment will experience loss, frustration, sadness and distress, that person may also experience humour (Marshall, 2001, 2011), creativity (Cahill et al, 2014a; Hazzan, 2016) and positive wellbeing (Woods, 2001). Indeed, many people who have dementia rate their quality of life more positively compared with how others (proxies) rate it (Thorgrimsen et al, 2003; Ettema et al, 2005; Cahill and Diaz-Ponce, 2017). In fact, with the appropriate interventions, drawn from the creative arts and humanities, such as art, dance, music (singing for the brain), reminiscence and aromatherapy (see Chapter Five), a person's strengths and retained abilities can be optimized. Yet the dominant discourse on dementia has virtually ignored the love, growth, purpose, participation and solidarity (Bartlett and O'Connor, 2010) that may also exist in life, despite a diagnosis of dementia.

The disability rights movement has been most successful in eliminating the pejorative language previously used to describe people with disabilities (Hughes, 2011), and words like 'retarded', 'handicapped', 'cripple', 'infirm' and 'imbecilic' are thankfully no longer in use. There is no reason why the language used today to describe people diagnosed with dementia cannot be changed and made less nihilistic and offensive. This will require education, particularly the training of journalists and other media staff, health service professionals, care workers, policy-makers, service planners and the public at large. A useful tool to promote more sensitive, inclusive language that is already available is the guidelines for language use developed by Alzheimer's Australia (2014). A useful platform to advance non-offensive language and to promote balanced messaging is through dementia awareness programmes. Emotive terminology, including words such as 'compassion', 'patients', 'journeys' and 'caregiver burden' need to be eliminated as they are divisive.

Finally, given how the word 'dementia' originates from the Latin word 'dement', meaning 'without mind', it is not surprising that 'dementia' has such negative connotations. Post (2000) contends that in the past 'dementia' was generally associated with 'syphilis', a very stigmatizing condition. Hughes (2011) claims that the word 'dementia' is an insulting, meaningless mess, given the diversity of symptoms the syndrome produces and the complexities contained in its pathology. He suggests how 'dementia' should be replaced with the expression 'acquired diffuse neurodegenerative cognitive dysfunction' (2011, p 17), which, in my view, is equally complex. The Japanese, visionary in their approach to dementia, having been the first nation to pioneer the concept of 'dementia champions' and 'dementia-friendly communities' (Rees, 2015; Imogen Blood and Associates, 2017), have removed the word dementia altogether from their vocabulary and replaced it with the words 'cognitive disorders'. But who amongst us wants to be labelled as having a 'disorder'? Perhaps a new word is needed for dementia that takes on board the diversity and complexity of the syndrome yet conveys the humanity and the uniqueness of the individual. This new word might bring the personhood and selfhood of the individual to the fore, reshape our thoughts and attitudes about dementia (George, 2010), and help us better 'connect to' rather than 'erect barriers against' the individual.

Conclusion

Conventional thinking (the standard paradigm) has constructed dementia as a cognitive brain disorder the symptoms of which include impairments in memory, thinking and learning, comprehension, communication, calculation, language and judgement – deficits arising due to the death of brain cells. This chapter has attempted to challenge conventional thinking and to show how dementia can be framed as a disability. Constructing dementia as a disability is not a new exercise but rather, what I have attempted to do is extend the debate by highlighting the opportunities such a construction can yield. A central theme underpinning the chapter is how dementia has remained under-represented in disability studies, and that there is a need for greater dialogue to take place between disability studies and dementia studies and between dementia activists and disability political activists. The chapter has critically reviewed three different models for understanding dementia – the biomedical, social and biopsychosocial. It has shown how dementia is well aligned with all three models since the syndrome is both (i) a health condition, (ii) a social construction and (iii) a neurological impairment influenced by a broad range of factors including biological, social, psychological, economic and cultural factors. The final part of the chapter has explored the way in which disability and people with disabilities are described in the CRPD. In so doing it has demonstrated why people living with dementia fall within the CRPD description of disability and therefore have full entitlement to each of its human rights. Much can be gained on the part of the individual, family member and health service professional by conceptualizing dementia as a disability. Not least is the fact that the rights set down in national and international legislation and treaties such as the CRPD can be used to challenge discriminatory attitudes, practices and policies that may deny people living with dementia their fundamental human rights. The chapter has therefore set the scene for Chapter Three, which will now advance to reviewing in greater detail the CRPD.

Summary of key points

- Apart from being a human rights issue, dementia is also a disability, although it rarely features in official reports on disability.
- Dementia has consistently remained under-reported in disability studies.
- Different models of disability can help us better understand dementia.
- The biomedical model offers insights into the causes of dementia, and heralds hope for a future cure.
- The social model places an emphasis on the way in which society constructs dementia and locates the problem of dementia as being outside the individual; it enables us to analyse oppressive and discriminatory policies and practice and focuses attention on human rights.
- The biopsychosocial model frames dementia within a health paradigm – the symptoms and behaviours of people who have dementia arise not just because of the disease process but are impacted on by a wide range of contextual factors (environmental and personal).

- The ICF tool underpinned by the biopsychosocial model of disability provides both a classification system and conceptual framework, and places a strong emphasis on the role the environment plays in the individual's experience of disability.
- The CRPD offers a useful framework for enhancing our understanding of disability and reflects the social model of disability.
- Compared with disability political activists the individual living with dementia confronts unique challenges when attempting to self advocate
- People living with dementia fit the CRPD's description of 'people with a disability' and are therefore entitled to claim each of the human rights set out in the Convention.
- Language is a powerful instrument for influencing attitudes and behaviours, and the language used to describe people living with dementia and their families needs to change.

Note

[1] The term 'handicap' was widely used in the past, and is still used today, in France.

THREE

Setting the context: The UN Convention on the Rights of Persons with Disabilities

> Too often, those living with disabilities have been seen as objects of embarrassment and at best of condescending pity and charity ... on paper they have enjoyed the same rights as others; in real life they have often been relegated to the margins and denied the opportunities that others take for granted. (Kofi Annan, 2006)

Introduction

In the opening chapters of this book I have argued that dementia is both a human rights issue (Chapter One) and a disability (Chapter Two), and in both chapters, reference was made to the CRPD. Since the CRPD is used as a compass for analysis in this book and is the common thread linking together the chapters, the purpose of this chapter is to provide an overview of its aims, principles and obligations. In this chapter I also identify the Articles selected for analysis in later chapters. Practical considerations including space limitations, along with my own personal evaluation of the relevance of these Articles to the life of the individual diagnosed with dementia and their family members, have determined this selection. At the outset it also needs to be acknowledged that the rights enshrined in the CRPD are all interrelated, indivisible and interdependent, which means that it would be very difficult to envisage one right, as, for example, the right to independent living, without considering other rights, as, for example, the right to legal capacity or the right to equality, autonomy, dignity and participation.

A key argument marshalled in this chapter is that the CRPD, underpinned by the social model of disability (Mental Health Foundation, 2015; Shakespeare et al, 2017), provides a solid springboard for the reframing of dementia as a human rights issue and for the emergence of social change in dementia policy and practice (McGettrick, 2014; Mental Health Foundation, 2015).

Notwithstanding its immense value as a treaty or formal agreement between states, when operationalized and applied to the lives of individuals who have dementia, the CRPD has some limitations and a later part of the chapter highlights these shortfalls and makes recommendations for change. The chapter concludes with an overview of some recent global and European developments that have helped reframe our thinking about dementia as a human rights issue.

An overview of the CRPD

After years of ongoing advocacy work and negotiations led by disability activists, disability people's organizations, academics, governments and non-government organizations (NGOs) (Schulze, 2010), the CRPD was finally adopted by the UN in 2006 and later ratified by the UN in 2009 (Mittler, 2016a). The CRPD is said to be a landmark treaty, since, despite differences in priorities and policies, the process leading to its development brought together international disabled people's constituencies that worked as equal partners in coalition with government bodies.

The CRPD did not enshrine new rights (Quinn, 2009; García-Iriarte et al, 2016); rather, it brought together disparate sets of human rights (civil, political, economic, social and cultural), and then, through non-discrimination principles (Quinn, 2009), explained how universal human rights can be made real in the context of disability. Thus, while the actual rights articulated in the CRPD were not new, the process was, since it involved the full and equal participation of many people with disabilities as key stakeholders and agents of change. These people with disabilities worked in partnership with politicians and senior officials at every stage in the process leading up to its adoption (Mittler, 2016a). In this way, the CRPD was significantly shaped and informed by people with disabilities along with disabled people's organizations (Schulze, 2010).

Worthy of note, too, is the fact that in the negotiations leading up to its adoption, there was a high level of participation from individuals with an intellectual disability, a group of people who in the past had been ignored (Mittler, 2016a). What is disappointing, however, is the absence of involvement of individuals living with dementia, their family members or representative organizations, in both the negotiations leading up to the development of the treaty, and later, as member(s) of the UN CRPD Committee, the specific body that monitors the implementation of the CRPD. This can in the future be rectified since Article 33, which refers to 'reporting guidelines', allows for civil society (including people with a disability) to be involved in their country's implementation and monitoring plans. This means that a person diagnosed with dementia, their family member or representative organizations can in the future become actively engaged in this process.

Aims of the CRPD

The broad aim of the CRPD (UN, 2006, p 4) was to 'promote, protect and ensure the full and equal enjoyment of human rights and fundamental freedoms by all persons with disabilities and to promote respect for their inherent dignity.' However, its scope was far reaching, since its commitment was to fundamentally change 'society's approach to understanding and responding to people with a disability' (Mental Health Foundation, 2015, p 11), and to eliminate differences arising in society between people with disabilities and those without disabilities. The CRPD was both a human rights treaty as well as a development tool – it required governments to implement approaches to ensure that persons with disabilities could enjoy full and equal participation in society (Schulze, 2010).

Unlike national human rights acts, the CRPD is not legally enforceable in court, although the UN CRPD Committee monitors and supports its implementation, and amongst other obligations, adjudicates on complaints lodged. In addition, the Office of the High Commissioner, led by the High Commissioner for Human Rights, who works to mainstream human rights throughout all UN programmes, supports the implementation of the CRPD (Nina Georgantzi, personal communication, 2017).

An essential starting point required by countries that have ratified (approved) the CRPD is the establishment of a focal point within governments, of which disabled people's organizations must be members. Ideally, this focal point should be in the Prime Minister's office with other focal points in other government departments (OHCHR, 2008). In signing what is referred to as the 'Optional Protocol', individuals and civil groups are entitled to raise complaints within the treaty body, provided they have already exhausted domestic solutions. Allowing the individual's voice to emerge through a complaints procedure like this is said to be particularly useful since it 'enables the raw edge of human experience to be expressed' (Quinn, 2009, p 246).

Principles

The core principles underpinning the CRPD and set down in Article 3 (UN, 2006, p 5) are:

- respect for inherent dignity, individual autonomy, including the freedom to make one's own choices and independence of persons
- non-discrimination
- full and effective participation and inclusion in society
- respect for differences and acceptance of people with disabilities as part of human diversity and humanity
- equality of opportunity
- accessibility
- equality between men and women
- respect for the evolving capacities of children with disabilities and respect for the right of children with disabilities to preserve their identities.

These principles are considered to be a 'legal reservoir', and provide the basis for change to legislation, policy and practice (Schulz, 2010). The principles cross cut each of the Articles and once ratified, States Parties (states or countries that have signed the Treaty) commit to complying with such principles (Mittler, 2016a). State Parties must also commit to complying with the obligations set out in the CRPD, and the section that follows details these particular obligations.

General obligations

The general obligations outlined in the CRPD are detailed in Article 4 (UN, 2006, pp 5-7) and must be fulfilled by countries that have ratified the CRPD. These include the protection and promotion of the human rights of persons with disabilities in all policies, the provision of accessible information to people with disabilities about aids, including devices and assistive technology (AT), and the promotion and training in human rights of all staff including professionals working in the field of disability. Amongst other issues, Article 4 requires the re-working of inconsistent legislation and where required, the adoption of new legislation (Quinn, 2009). Schulz (2010, p 50) summarizes these obligations to include as follows:

- 'Adopting legislative administrative and other appropriate measures for the implementation of rights.
- Modifying or abolishing laws, regulations, customs or practices that might be discriminatory.
- Including in all relevant policies and programmes the protection and promotion of the human rights of persons with disabilities.
- Refraining from any action or practice inconsistent with the Convention and ensuring that public authorities and institutions conform to the Convention.
- Undertaking or promoting research and development as defined in Article 2 of the Convention.
- Providing accessible information of persons with disabilities about mobility aids, devices and assistive technologies.
- Promoting the training of professionals and staff working with persons with disabilities in the rights enshrined in the CRPD.
- Taking all measures to abolish discrimination against people with disability.'

Paradigm shift

The CRPD is said to reflect a major paradigm shift in contemporary disability discourse (Quinn, 2010; Mittler, 2016a). Rather than seeing a person as a passive object of charity, the treaty regards the individual with a disability as an active holder of human rights. Its mantra 'nothing about us without us' (Charlton, 1998), adopted from the Disability Rights movement, reminds us of the central role people with disabilities have themselves played in developing the treaty. This mantra has also been enshrined into a binding provision in Article 33 that explicitly states that 'persons with disabilities and their representative organizations, shall be involved and participate fully in the monitoring process' (UN, 2006, p 25). The CRPD holds as a starting premise the fact that all human beings are born equal, and possess certain inalienable rights. It places obligations on governments and civil society to respect, protect and promote the human rights of persons with disabilities. It urges governments and civil society to take action to remove all obstacles and barriers that create disability. The Articles are said to present a challenge to governments, service commissioners and practitioners who must assess how supports and practices within countries comply with obligations to promote rights (Stainton and Clare, 2012).

Terminology

Ratifying the CRPD and its implications

Earlier reference was made to the general obligations required from countries that have 'ratified' the CRPD. The distinction between 'signing' and 'ratifying' the CRPD is important since signing merely means that a country has entered into an agreement to respect various obligations set down in the CRPD and must submit to the Committee a report that guarantees rights on the development and implementation of public policy, whilst ratification means that a country has entered into agreement in international law to convert the CRPD's principles into both policy and practice. Ratification also requires countries to adhere to guidelines set out in Article 33, and to regularly report to the UN CRPD Committee, established to oversee its implementation (WHO and The World Bank, 2011).

As mentioned, the CRPD was first adopted by the UN in 2006 and ratified by the UN in 2009. In 2010 it was ratified by the European Union (EU). The EU's ratification is significant as it made the EU the first supranational government to ratify a human rights treaty (ENNHRI, 2016). As at December 2016, the CRPD had been ratified by 172 countries and signed by 160 (UN, 2016).[1] Ireland is the only country in Europe that to date has not ratified the CRPD. Almost a decade ago, Quinn (2009) noted that a reason for this is that Ireland's legislation on legal capacity required updating. Although new mental health legislation (Assisted Decision-Making [Capacity] Act 2015) was passed in Ireland in December 2015, now at the time of writing, ratification of the CRPD by Ireland has still not taken place, which leaves Irish people who have a disability, including those living with dementia, exceptionally vulnerable.

Immediate implementation versus progressive realization

Other terms important to our understanding of the operationalization of the CRPD include 'immediate implementation' versus 'progressive realization' of human rights. Quinn (2009, p 247) refers to 'obligations of result', that is, those human rights that must take *immediate effect*, versus 'obligations of conduct' or those human rights that can be *achieved over time*. In his view there is a bias against enforcing 'rights of conduct' such as economic, social and cultural rights, since they are resource-intensive. In contrast, enforcing 'rights of result' such as civil and political rights, including the right to legal capacity, must be implemented immediately.

In the context of social, economic and cultural rights or 'rights of conduct', countries that have ratified the CRPD must provide concrete evidence of *progressive realization*. This means that they need only demonstrate that they are doing everything within their power and available resources to ensure that people with disabilities can enjoy their human rights as quickly as possible (EHRC, 2010). Progressive realization also requires States Parties to show a national plan of action over a given period of time – once in the first two years and thereafter every four years (Mittler, 2016a). These implementation plans must identify parties responsible for the plan, including people with disabilities, and outline the action taken or planned on being taken under each Article. Countries are also expected to submit detailed progress reports to the UN CRPD Committee.

General Comments

General Comments provide contextual interpretation of the abstract rights contained in treaties, and provide guidance on how rights should be implemented in practice and what obligations they generate for States Parties. Although strictly speaking General Comments are not legally binding, they are still considered to have authoritative status (Nina Georgantzi, personal communication, 2017).[2]

Articles in the CRPD

A classification system

The CRPD is the first human rights treaty adopted in the 21st century and is said to provide both a 'philosophical framework' and 'language' to individuals who experience injustice and discrimination (Quinn, 2009). It contains 50 Articles, which cover a broad range of human rights topics, including rights to education, equality, independent living and accessibility. In her thought-provoking book, *From rhetoric to action: Implementing the UN Convention on the Rights of Persons with Disabilities*, Flynn (2011) provides a useful typology for the classification of these Articles that she claims are underpinned by four broad themes: (i) equality, (ii) autonomy, (iii) participation and (iv) solidarity (see Figure 3.1).

Figure 3.1: Key themes identified by Flynn in the CRPD

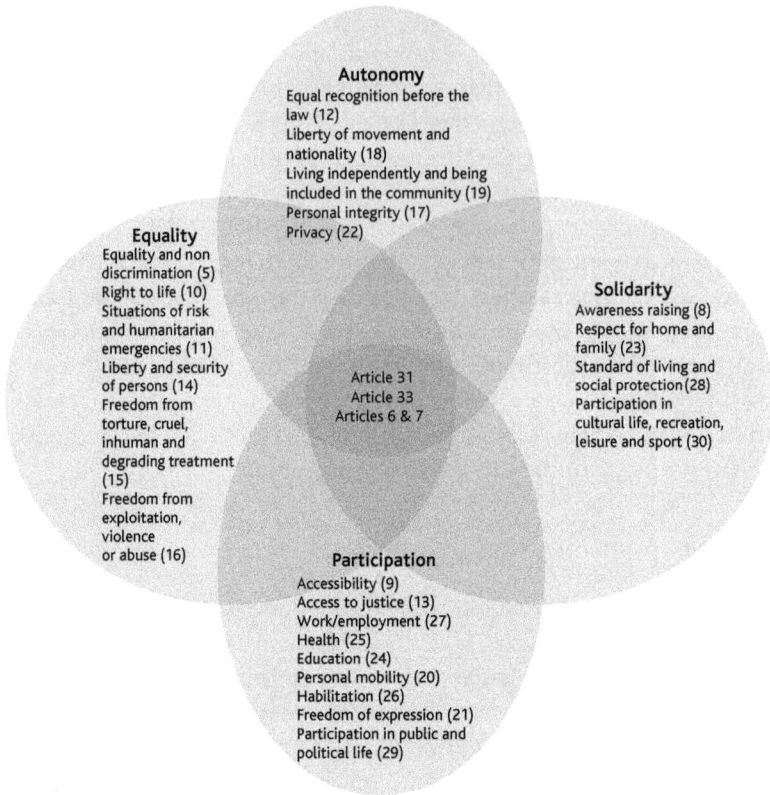

Autonomy
Equal recognition before the
law (12)
Liberty of movement and
nationality (18)
Living independently and being
included in the community (19)
Personal integrity (17)
Privacy (22)

Equality
Equality and non
discrimination (5)
Right to life (10)
Situations of risk
and humanitarian
emergencies (11)
Liberty and security
of persons (14)
Freedom from
torture, cruel,
inhuman and
degrading treatment
(15)
Freedom from
exploitation,
violence
or abuse (16)

Solidarity
Awareness raising (8)
Respect for home and
family (23)
Standard of living and
social protection (28)
Participation in
cultural life, recreation,
leisure and sport (30)

Article 31
Article 33
Articles 6 & 7

Participation
Accessibility (9)
Access to justice (13)
Work/employment (27)
Health (25)
Education (24)
Personal mobility (20)
Habilitation (26)
Freedom of expression (21)
Participation in public and
political life (29)

Source: Flynn (2011) p 14.

Equality: refers to the fact that everyone is equal before the law, and disabled people have exactly the same rights to freedom, dignity, equality and respect on a par with everyone else (Flynn, 2011). This approach challenges belief systems that set some people apart from others on the basis of different attributes, 'or that deprive some sorts of human beings of any standing, or that give no standing at all to individual persons as individuals' (Jones, 2000, p 214). Articles in the CRPD that cover these broad themes include Article 5 (equality and non-discrimination), Article 10 (the right to life), Article 14 (the right to liberty and security) and Article 15 (freedom from torture or cruel treatment). Most importantly, the CRPD considers that everyone has a right to legal capacity or to hold and execute legal rights, and everyone, irrespective of disability, is considered equal before the law. In the context of the everyday life of the individual living with dementia and their family members, the right to legal capacity has very profound ramifications. This topic is explored in much greater detail in Chapters Four and Seven of this book.

Autonomy: known in Greek history as 'self rule' (Welford et al, 2010, p 1233), and defined as 'making decisions and choices and directing one's own life' (Kane, 2001, p 298) or the 'right to self determination' (Nuffield Council on Bioethics, 2009, p 26), autonomy is said to be integral to human dignity as reflected in the CRPD's Preamble core principles. These principles include 'respect for inherent dignity individual autonomy including the freedom to make one's own choices, and independence of persons' (UN, 2006, p 5). Inextricably linked to this theme of autonomy is the notion of privacy, the fact that nobody with a disability, irrespective of their living arrangements, should be subjected to having their private lives interfered with. The important concepts of choice, control and independence also lie at the very core of this same theme of autonomy (Murphy and Welford, 2012; OECD, 2015). Whilst traditional accounts of autonomy have tended to place an unprecedented emphasis on rationality (see Nuffield Council on Bioethics, 2009), in this book, the notion of 'relational autonomy' is explored. This approach reflects a recognition that 'respect for autonomy must involve others taking active steps to act as advocates and to try to promote [that person's] autonomy' (Nuffield Council on Bioethics, p 27). Examples of Articles in the CRPD which reflect this theme include Article 12 (equal recognition before the law), Article 19 (living independently and being included in the community) and Article 22 (privacy).

Participation: builds on components of the ICF model of health and disability (WHO, 2001) discussed in the previous chapter, and on the premise that all human beings, irrespective of difference, including disability, have the right to participate in every aspect of public, political, social, economic and cultural life. Closely associated with the concept of participation is the right of people with a disability to have equal access to a choice of community services including transport, housing and information (Flynn, 2011). It also includes their rights to access a wide range of in-home, residential and other community services, including the personal assistance required to support inclusion and living in the community. Examples of Articles in the CRPD which reflect this theme include Article 9 (accessibility), Article 25 (health) and Article 26 (habilitation and rehabilitation).

Solidarity: refers to social citizenship and the fact that we are all interdependent and have responsibilities within our families and within society (Hughes, 2011). The Nuffield Council on Bioethics (2009, p 29) describes solidarity as the notion '... that we are all fellow travellers and that we have duties to support and help each other and particularly those who cannot readily support themselves.' In accordance with Flynn's (2011) typology, the Articles in the CRPD that reflect this theme of solidarity include awareness raising (Article 8), respect for home and family (Article 23), standard of living, social protection (Article 28), and the right to participate in recreational, cultural leisure time and sporting activities (Article 29). In later chapters of this book, several of these broad themes will be revisited.

CRPD Articles particularly relevant to people living with dementia and their family members

Table 3.1 details those Articles in the CRPD chosen for critical review in this book. They have been selected on the basis that they are particularly relevant to the lives of individuals experiencing the symptoms of dementia, their family members, health service professionals, policy-makers and other key stakeholders. Townsend (2006, p 166) contends that, 'Violations are not only those that end life or involve extreme abuse the scale of which is assembled in statistical handbooks, but also those that affront human dignity and identity which are unrecorded.' Accordingly, whilst the human rights chosen for critical review in this book reflect in many cases more subtle topics, it is hoped that the range of rights chosen is sufficiently broad to give the reader a flavour of the type of everyday freedoms that may be denied to people because of a diagnosis of dementia.

Table 3.1 CRPD Articles particularly relevant to dementia and selected for review

Article	Title	Standards/rights covered
Article 3	General principles	a) Respect for inherent dignity, individual autonomy including the freedom to make one's own choices and independence of persons b) Non-discrimination c) Full and effective participation and inclusion in society d) Respect for difference and acceptance of persons with disability as part of human diversity and humanity e) Equality of opportunity f) Accessibility g) Equality between men and women h) Respect for the evolving capacities of children with disabilities and respect for the right of children with disabilities to preserve their identities
Article 4	General obligations	1. States Parties undertake to ensure and promote the full realization of all human rights and fundamental freedoms for all person with disabilities without discrimination of any kind on the basis of disability. To this end States Parties undertake: a) To adopt all appropriate legislative, administrative and other measures for the implementation of the rights recognized in the present Convention b) To take all appropriate measures, including legislation, to modify or abolish existing laws, regulations, customs and practices that constitute discrimination against persons with disabilities c) To take into account the protection and promotion of the human rights of persons with disabilities in all policies h) To provide accessible information to persons with disabilities about mobility aids, devices and assistive technologies, including new technologies as well as other forms of assistance, support services and facilities i) To promote the training of professionals and staff working with persons with disabilities in the rights recognized in this Convention so as to better provide the assistance and services guaranteed by those rights 2. With regard to economic, social and cultural rights each State Party undertakes to take measures to the maximum of its available resources and where needed, within the framework of international cooperation, with a view to achieving progressively the full realization of these rights without prejudice to those obligations contained in the present Convention that are immediately applicable according to international law.

Article	Title	Standards/rights covered
Article 5	Equality and non-discrimination	1. States Parties recognize that all persons are equal before and under the law and are entitled without any discrimination to the equal protection and equal benefit of the law. 2. States Parties shall prohibit all discrimination on the basis of disability and guarantee to persons with disabilities equal and effective legal protection against discrimination on all grounds.
Article 9	Accessibility	1. To enable persons with disabilities to live independently and participate fully in all aspects of life, States Parties shall take appropriate measures to ensure persons with disabilities access on an equal basis with others to the physical environment, to transportation, to information and communications, including information and communications technologies and systems and to other facilities and services open or provided to the public, both in urban and in rural areas. These measures which shall include the identification and elimination of obstacles and barriers to accessibility shall apply to inter alia.
Article 12	Equal recognition before the law	1. States Parties reaffirm that persons with disabilities have the right to recognition everywhere as persons before the law. 2. States Parties shall recognize that persons with disabilities enjoy legal capacity on an equal basis with others in all aspects of life . 3. States Parties shall take appropriate measures to provide access by persons with disabilities to the support they may require in exercising their legal capacity.
Article 15	Freedom from torture or cruel, inhuman or degrading treatment or punishment	1. No one shall be subjected to torture or to cruel, inhuman or degrading treatment or punishment. In particular, no one shall be subjected without his or her free consent to medical or scientific experimentation. 2. States Parties shall take all effective legislative, administrative, judicial or other measures to prevent persons with disabilities, on an equal basis with others, from being subjected to torture or cruel, inhuman or degrading treatment or punishment.
Article 19	Living independently and being included in the community	1. States Parties to this Convention recognize the equal right of all persons with disabilities to live in the community, with choices equal to others, and shall take effective and appropriate measures to facilitate full enjoyment by persons with disabilities of this right and their full inclusion and participation in the community including by ensuring that: a) Persons with disabilities have the opportunity to choose their place of residence and where and with whom they live on an equal basis with others and are not obliged to live in a particular living arrangement b) Persons with disabilities have access to a range of in-home, residential and other community support services including personal assistance necessary to support living and inclusion in the community and to prevent isolation or segregation from the community c) Community services and facilities for the general population are available on an equal basis to persons with disabilities and are responsive to their needs.

Article	Title	Standards/rights covered
Article 22	Respect for privacy	1. No person with disabilities, regardless of place of residence or living arrangements, shall be subjected to arbitrary or unlawful interference with his or her privacy, family, home or correspondence or other types of communication or to unlawful attacks on his or her honour and reputation. Persons with disabilities have the right to the protection of the law against such interference or attacks. 2. States Parties shall protect the privacy of personal, health and rehabilitation information of persons with disabilities on an equal basis with others.
Article 25	Health	1. States Parties recognize that persons with disabilities have the right to the enjoyment of the highest attainable standard of health without discrimination on the basis of disability. States Parties shall take all appropriate measures to ensure access for persons with disabilities to health services that are gender-sensitive, including health-related rehabilitation. In particular, States Parties shall: a) Provide persons with disabilities with the same range, quality and standard of free or affordable health care and programmes as provided to other persons, including in the area of sexual and reproductive health and population-based public health programmes b) Provide those health services needed by persons with disabilities specifically because of their disabilities, including early identification and intervention as appropriate, and services designed to minimize and prevent further disabilities including among children and older persons c) Provide these services as close as possible to people's own communities, including in rural areas d) Require health professionals to provide care of the same quality to persons with disabilities as to others, including on the basis of free and informed consent by, inter alia, raising awareness of the human rights, dignity, autonomy and needs of persons with disabilities through training and the promulgation of ethical standards for public and private healthcare
Article 26	Habilitation and rehabilitation	1. States Parties shall take effective and appropriate measures including through peer support, to enable persons with disabilities to attain and maintain maximum independence, full physical, mental, social and vocational ability and full inclusion and participation in all aspects of life. To that end States Parties shall organize, strengthen and extend comprehensive habilitation and rehabilitation services and programmes, particularly in the areas of health, employment, education and social services, in such a way that these services and programmes: a) Begin at the earliest possible stage and are based on multidisciplinary assessment of individual needs and strengths b) Support participation and inclusion in the community and all aspects of society, are voluntary and are available to persons with disabilities as close as possible to their own communities, including in rural areas.

Article	Title	Standards/rights covered
Article 30	Participation in cultural life, recreation, leisure and sport	1. States Parties recognize the right of persons with disabilities to take part on an equal basis with others in cultural life, and shall take all appropriate measures to ensure that persons with disabilities: a) Enjoy access to cultural materials in accessible formats b) Enjoy access to television programmes, films, theatre and other cultural activities in accessible formats c) Enjoy access to places for cultural performances or services such as theatres, museums, cinemas, libraries and tourism services, and as far as possible enjoy access to monuments and sites of national cultural importance 2. States Parties shall take appropriate measures to enable persons with disabilities to have the opportunity to develop and utilize their creative, artistic and intellectual potential, not only for their own benefit, but also for the enrichment of society
Article 33	National implementation and monitoring	1. States Parties, in accordance with their system of organization, shall designate one or more focal points within government for matters relating to the implementation of the present Convention, and shall give due consideration to the establishment or designation of a coordination mechanism within government to facilitate related action indifferent sectors and at different levels. 2. States Parties shall, in accordance with their legal and administrative systems, maintain, strengthen, designate or establish within the State Party, a framework, including one or more independent mechanisms, as appropriate, to promote, protect and monitor implementation of the present Convention. When designating or establishing such a mechanism, States Parties shall take into account the principles relating to the statues and functioning of national institutions for protection and promotion of human rights. 3. Civil society, in particular persons with disabilities and their representative organizations, shall be involved and participate fully in the monitoring process.

Source: UN (2006) Convention on the Rights of Persons with Disabilities (CRPD), New York: United Nations. Reprinted with the permission of the United Nations.
Note: Not all Articles or part Articles are included in the table.

A critique of the CRPD

Although Mittler (2012) has argued that the CRPD is relevant to the life of the individual diagnosed with dementia and their family members and others (Eilionóir Flynn, personal communication, 2016), she claims that the treaty was intended to target persons living with dementia; the absence of recognition of dementia as a disability in disability activism (as discussed in Chapter Two) is again reflected in the way nobody with dementia or their representative organizations (such as Alzheimer societies or the ADI) participated in the original negotiations, leading up to the development and adoption of the CRPD. It is therefore not surprising that when the CRPD is used to interrogate dementia policy and practice, it has some limitations.

For example, the wording of Article 15, 'freedom from torture or cruel, inhuman or degrading treatment or punishment' and protection from 'medical or scientific experimentation', fails to explicitly protect the unique rights of the individual with a severe dementia, including their right to be protected from excessive and inappropriate use of chemical and physical restraints. Although it could be argued that Article 17 (protecting the integrity of the person) and Article 25 (health) address these rights, a General Comment on Article 15 would provide for the more specific challenges the individual living with a more severe dementia may confront.

Article 19, which refers to the rights of people with disabilities to choose their place of residence and to have the personal assistance necessary to support living, has profound implications for the individual diagnosed with dementia. Yet the scope of this Article is significantly undermined by the 'progressive realization' clause embedded in Article 4(2). Regarding the fulfilment of social, cultural and economic rights this stipulates that 'each State party undertakes to take measures [only] to the maximum of its available resources and, where needed, within the framework of international cooperation with a view to achieve progressively the full realization of these rights ...' (UN, 2006, p 6).

Article 19, which refers to independent living is also complex as it includes elements of civil and political rights as well as social rights. For example, whilst the provision of community services is a social right, concepts of choice and non-discrimination embedded in this same Article are linked to civil rights including autonomy. If Article 19 was considered only a civil right, it would be immediately enforceable, but because it is seen as a social right, the principle of 'progressive realization', as explained earlier, applies (Nina Georgantzi, personal communication, 2017). The other limitation of Article 19 is that it is hugely weighted in favour of deinstitutionalization. An unintended consequence here may be that a small minority of people diagnosed with dementia may be forced to remain at home in the community, when, in fact, they themselves might favour long-term residential care (OECD, 2015).

The CRPD has also been written primarily to promote the rights of people with disabilities living in the 'community'. This means that across the Articles there is a notable absence of reference to issues relevant to the lives of individuals living in 'care homes' or 'nursing homes', such as their right not to be evicted from residential care settings as a result of 'behaviours that challenge' or their right to end-of-life care services in residential care settings including hospice/palliative care services.

Although it is noted that the global dementia community, including representative advocacy bodies, have, until recently, shown limited interest in availing themselves of the opportunities made possible by the CRPD (Mittler, 2015; Williamson, 2015; Mental Health Foundation, 2015), possibly because dementia tends not to be viewed as a disability (Shakespeare et al, 2017), this trend is changing (Rees, 2015; DAI, 2016), and the final part of the chapter advances to highlighting some recent political events that have helped highlight the importance of the CRPD as an advocacy tool for the individual diagnosed with dementia, and that have helped to further reframe dementia as a human rights concern.

Recent political developments

Charter of rights for people with dementia and their carers in Scotland

Scotland leads the world in the area of dementia policy and practice, having, in 2002, been the first nation to establish a dementia working group (an advocacy group comprising people living with dementia and established to raise awareness of dementia), making dementia a national health priority in 2007, setting national targets for improving diagnostic rates in 2008 (Scotland's national dementia strategy [2013-2016], see Scottish Government, 2013), and since 2013, being the only country in the world, as far as I am aware, to now guarantee 12 months post-diagnostic services to its people. Not surprisingly, therefore, it was Scotland that in 2009 produced the first Charter of Rights for people with dementia and their carers, a document that mirrors the human rights outlined in the CRPD and in other international instruments (SPCPGOA, 2009). The Charter, which is said to have informed the Scottish dementia strategy (Gráinne McGettrick, personal communication, 2016), also drew on mental health legislation and human rights instruments, to improve outcomes for people living with dementia and their family members. Its aim was to empower the individual and family members by guaranteeing them the fullest possible realization of their human rights. The Charter was important politically as it brought together members of the Scottish Parliament and civil society, including those living with dementia, their family members and their representatives, and involved the establishment of the Scottish Parliament's Cross-Party Group on Alzheimer's disease.

Since its development other countries, including Ireland have also developed their own Charters (ASI, 2016).

Thematic briefing for the first WHO ministerial conference

Another important indicator of this gradually evolving rights-based movement in dementia is reflected in WHO's (2015a) thematic briefing paper, *Ensuring a human rights-based approach for people living with dementia*, prepared for its first ministerial conference on dementia held in Geneva in 2015. Although pithy and to the point, politically, this paper is strategic as in it WHO explicitly commits to ensuring that a rights-based framework is applied to all global action on dementia, and that all measures related to dementia, including legislation and policy, be linked to human rights standards. In the past WHO had been critiqued for its over-medicalization of dementia as, for example, in its report, *Dementia: A public health priority* (WHO, 2012), where it was claimed that undue emphasis was placed on disease, burden, risks, treatments, costs and the needs of carers (Thomas and Milligan, 2015). This concise paper that draws on international case studies reveals a broadening in focus of WHO's conceptualization of dementia with a more nuanced emphasis now placed on human rights, including equity, empowerment and legality.

Dementia rights and the social model of disability

A third indicator of this gradually evolving rights-based movement in dementia policy and practice is reflected in the paper, *Dementia rights and the social model of disability* (Mental Health Foundation, 2015), a provocative discussion paper, written and overseen by individuals living with dementia, disability activists, legal experts, academics and representatives from government and NGOs, and intended to influence policy-makers and practitioners. In the paper, the social model of dementia is pitched against the biomedical model, as two stand-alone entities. The social model is revered as the way forward as it has the potential to lead dementia discourse in new directions, influence what is talked about and essentially who does this talking (Guleria and Curtice, 2016). However, none of the shortcomings of the social model in the context of its application to the individual who has dementia are discussed. The discussion paper incites organizations to have their policies and practices evaluated against human rights standards and principles (Mental Health Foundation Report, 2015).

From a policy perspective, a useful aspect of this paper is Table 4 (p 19), where the principles of participation, accountability, non-discrimination, empowerment and legality (PANEL) used most often in social justice work are applied to interrogate dementia policy and the policy-making process (see Table 3.2).

Table 3.2: Using the PANEL principles to operationalize a human rights-based approach in dementia practice, the key questions (macro level)

The PANEL or human rights-based approach and key questions	
Participation Everyone has the right to participate in decisions that affect their lives	Are people with dementia involved in the process policy? Have any barriers to their involvement been identified and addressed?
Accountability Effective monitoring of human rights standards and remedies for breaches	Who is responsible for the process/policy? Is there a way of assessing whether they have carried out their responsibilities? Is there a mechanism to hold them accountable?
Non-discrimination and equality All forms of discrimination in the realization of rights are prohibited, prevented and eliminated, with priority given to the most vulnerable	Have individuals and groups of people with dementia been identified as being vulnerable to human rights breaches? How might the policy impact on people with dementia? What can be done to be inclusive of people with dementia/lessen the negative impact of the policy?
Empowerment Individuals and communities should understand their rights and be supported to participate in the development of policy and practices that affect their lives	What information will people with dementia who are affected by the policy/decision need in order to be able to effectively influence the decision?
Legality of rights Recognition of rights that are legally enforceable entitlements (linked to national and international law)	Is the approach explicitly grounded in human rights law? Does it follow the relevant principles of human rights law? If there is relevant legislation does it comply? Is the legal framework explicitly stated so that rights holders can use it to bolster their claims?

Source: Adapted from ASI (2013), the SHRC (2015) and the Mental Health Foundation (2015)

However, what is missing is information or guidelines about how exactly these PANEL principles can be applied in practice to address service inequities, challenge poor practice, interrogate quality of care and improve practice (Kelly and Innes, 2012). This is a task I have set myself in Chapter six of this book.

ADI's adoption of a human rights approach to dementia

Yet a further indicator of the groundswell support for framing dementia as a human rights issue is reflected in the ADI's formal adoption in 2016 of a human rights-based approach to dementia policy (Shakespeare et al, 2017). In recent years, the ADI has been working in close partnership with the DAI, and in August 2016, the two organizations provided briefings to the UN CRPD Committee. Their requests were to ensure that the resources of the UN would be extended and used to monitor the extent to which people living with dementia are included in a country's implementation of the CRPD.

This appeal and its timing was no doubt strategic, given that WHO's new global action plan on dementia, strongly embedded in human rights principles, was issued in September 2016 (Rees, 2017). It may be no surprise, then, that this authoritative policy document makes numerous references to human rights and to the CRPD. Although it is difficult to know exactly what factors have influenced the rights based focus in the document, it is likely that the DAI's report submitted to the UN CRPD Committee (Shakespeare et al, 2017), along with earlier documents and events discussed here, have had a significant influence.

WHO's global action plan on the public health response to dementia

This global action plan, which was endorsed by the World Assembly in May 2017, is considered to be one of the most transparent and business-like documents in respect of chronic disease (Rees, 2017). Developed to improve the lives of people living with dementia and their families and to reduce the impact of dementia, both at an individual and population level (WHO, 2016), the plan details seven priority action areas and in relation to each, identifies clear targets for countries to reach over a given period. Although the plan is not legal and WHO cannot force member states to commit, it does require ministries or government departments in each of its 194 member states to report to WHO on a regular basis (Rees, 2017). Civil society, including the ADI and its members, need to hold countries and members to account and intervene when they do not perform (Marc Wortmann, personal communication, 2017).

The global action plan is underpinned by seven cross-cutting principles including those of empowerment, engagement and equity. In fact, the first of these seven principles, 'the human rights of people with dementia' explicitly states that [all]: 'Policies, plans, legislation, programmes, interventions and actions should be sensitive to the needs, expectations and human rights of people with dementia consistent with the Convention on the rights of persons with disabilities and other international and regional human rights instruments' (WHO, 2016, p 6). The action plan is most important as it provides countries around the world with a clear vision for future policy development and later chapters of this book will return to a more in-depth analysis of this action plan on dementia.

Conclusion

This chapter has provided a brief overview of the CRPD, describing its aims and principles, and detailing the specific obligations required of countries that have signed or ratified the Treaty. It has outlined the typology developed by Flynn (2011) to classify the key themes of equality, autonomy, participation and solidarity that straddle the rights contained in the CRPD: themes which will thread through later chapters of this book. The chapter has also introduced the reader to the selection of Articles which will be critically reviewed by me in Chapters Four and Five and to the PANEL principles which will be further explored in Chapter Six. In this chapter I have also provided a brief critique of the CRPD pointing to those Articles particularly relevant to dementia, that may in the future warrant General Comments. The final part of the chapter has advanced to a discussion and critique of a selection of recent publications on the topic of human rights and dementia. These papers reflect a shift in the dominant discourse, and show how a rights-based movement in dementia policy and practice is gradually gaining momentum. The chapter has shown that the CRPD offers a unique opportunity to reframe dementia as a social disability and human rights issue (Mental Health Foundation, 2015). Importantly, the CRPD offers people living with dementia the potential for legal protection (Article 12), entitlement to services (Article 19) and to interactions with service providers 'trained' in human rights (Article 4). Using the CRPD as a tool to re-cast dementia allows for a new and exciting dialogue to emerge, where the framing of dementia is no longer characterized by stigma, fear and exclusion, but rather, where the individual with dementia is viewed as a legitimate part of mainstream society (McGettrick, 2014). The new discourse reflects a shift in the balance of power and control, where the person can have agency and can be encouraged and supported to participate in the policy process (Mental Health Foundation, 2015).

Summary of key points

- Dementia is a disability, and because of this, the CRPD has direct relevance to the lives of all people living with dementia and their families.
- Whilst people with a disability played an active role in the discussions and negotiations leading up to the adoption of the CRPD, nobody living with dementia, their family members or their representative organizations were active participants in these discussions or negotiations.
- Drawing on Article 33, people living with dementia, their family members and/or representative organizations including advocacy groups have the opportunity now to become actively involved and participate fully in their countries' monitoring and implementation of the CRPD.
- The CRPD is a useful tool for reframing dementia as a human rights issue and for providing a language and a philosophical framework to those who experience injustices and discrimination.
- The Articles within the CRPD present a challenging agenda for governments, policy-makers and practitioners.
- A slowly evolving rights-based movement, led primarily by dementia activists, is beginning to gain traction around the world.
- The last two years have witnessed this rights-based movement gaining significant momentum.
- WHO's global action plan on dementia (2016), which makes explicit reference to the CRPD, is a policy document firmly embedded in human rights-based principles.
- Policy-makers, health service professionals, care workers, service commissioners, service regulators, researchers, people living with dementia and their family members and the public at large need to familiarise themselves with the CRPD.
- Policy-makers, health service professionals, care workers, service commissioners, service regulators, researchers, people living with dementia and their family members and the public at large need to familiarise themselves with the global action plan on dementia (WHO, 2016).

Note

[1] For an updated list, see https://treaties.un.org/Pages/ViewDetails.aspx?src=TREATY&mtdsg_no=IV-15&chapter=4&clang=_en

[2] See www.institut-fuer-menschenrechte.de/en/topics/development/frequently-asked-questions/9-what-are-general-comments/; www2.ohchr.org/english/bodies/treaty/glossary.htm; www.ohchr.org/EN/HRBodies/Pages/TBGeneralComments.aspx

PART TWO

Using a human rights lens to interrogate policy and practice

FOUR

The right to a good quality of life at home and in the community

In 2006 I had a mild head injury which resulted in my seeing three doctors and taking a Mini-Mental State Examination test and other neurological testing. I was told by my neurologist that I had a head injury; however, the other two doctors suggested I may have Alzheimer's disease which could be brought about sooner because of my head injury. I *struggled* for a few more years and was informed there is no definitive test for Alzheimer's. I subsequently took another opinion in 2011 due to my inability to cope and was diagnosed with early onset Alzheimer's in 2012 at the age of 62 while I was busy working and planning my retirement. It was like a slow realisation that a creeping fog had descended on your life and it was there for good....

A flurry of visits to the doctor and the consultant followed, as I tried to come to terms with the diagnosis, but there was yet another blow to come. More bad news; the threshold age for early onset Alzheimer's support is 65. For anyone diagnosed with early onset dementia-related illnesses before their 65th birthday, *there is nothing, and I mean nothing at all; no support services, nowhere to go, no one to give you advice or tips on how to proceed.* For me, having spent my adult life campaigning for human rights, this was inconceivable. *I couldn't believe that because of a random number, I would be ignored.* Worse still, refused all help and services. But I didn't have the strength or will to fight it. I retreated. I felt helpless for the first time in my life, no plan, no ideas and no strategies.

Those first few months were spent grappling with heartbreak, and although I still felt my career and voluntary work defined who I was, and how I was thought of in the community, I was too ashamed to mention my condition to anyone. I was more than aware of the stigma associated with it. I felt there was nobody to turn to except the internet. I wish somebody had been there to hold my hand

and explain to me Alzheimer's is not just about memory, that it impacts our ability to accomplish daily tasks, that it hinders our thinking process and the horrendous pain that agitation brings, not just to me, but to my family. *I would have loved somebody to give me advice on telling my family*, and if there were any supports available for them. The right to information is fundamental to participation in society as a person with dementia.

Eventually, I got the courage to seek help and start telling people I had the condition. I looked up research being carried out through Trinity College which led to me to The Alzheimer Society of Ireland and the newly formed Irish Dementia Working Group. Until I reached out and got help all I could see was the deepest grief imaginable, but somehow, after I told people, I could see some light. Thankfully I was able to participate in cognitive rehabilitation through Trinity College and The Alzheimer Society of Ireland; this gave me some valuable tools and strategies. Four years ago I would not leave the house; now I'm travelling with assistance, driving (having passed my test) and living life with support from family, friends and The Alzheimer Society. I am travelling all over the world speaking about dementia and campaigning for rights. (Helen Rochford-Brennan, Chairperson of the European Dementia Working Group, 2016; emphasis added)

When people think about dementia and human rights, they tend to reflect on the big ticket issues such as abuse scandals in nursing homes or hospital 'Do Not Resuscitate' policies, and not on the everyday affronts to human rights the individual living with dementia often experiences as this opening narrative illustrates, and as a person attempts to exercise choice and control over matters critical to their own independence, autonomy, health and wellbeing.

This chapter aims to expand public discourse on dementia as a rights-based issue, by exploring a number of rights, usually taken for granted, indeed, generally perceived as fundamental to those of us not cognitively disabled, but often restricted or denied to a person living with dementia. In particular, and with reference to the CRPD, the chapter addresses the individual's rights to:

- be treated equally before the law
- early diagnosis and its ethical and sensitive disclosure

- rehabilitation/reablement based on a multidisciplinary assessment and
- live well in the community with access to a range of support services including personal assistance.

With rising prevalence rates and the numbers of people affected by dementia likely to reach 135 million by 2050 (ADI, 2015), and as the world eagerly awaits a cure, governments around the world, alongside clinicians, researchers, academics, Alzheimer's associations and the wider dementia community, are working hard to develop national dementia strategies designed to reduce public expenditure and improve quality of care (Fortinsky and Downs, 2014). However, to what extent do these strategies/plans actually take cognizance of people's human rights (Kelly and Innes, 2012)? Given how some of us, because of our age, are at risk of getting dementia, and all of us probably at some stage in our lives will come into close contact with a person who has dementia, these are important questions to consider. By using the CRPD as a prism for analysis, this chapter aims to explore these topics particularly as they relate to people living with dementia at home, in the community.

Although, as noted by Brooker (2004), the dominant and most influential discourse on dementia has up until recently centred on human needs and personhood (Kitwood, 1997a) and not on human rights (Mental Health Foundation, 2015), the idea that people living with dementia have human rights is not new (King's Fund Centre, 1986; Cantley and Bowes, 2004; Gilliard et al, 2005; ADI, 2011; Brooker and Latham, 2016), yet a rights-based approach has rarely been explicitly applied to challenge the discrimination, marginalization and exclusionary practices and policies many people living with dementia experience (Kelly and Innes, 2012; Mittler, 2015; Bartlett, 2016; WHO, 2016). This may be because, traditionally, human rights tended to focus on capacity, rationality and decision-making ability (Bartlett and O'Connor, 2007; Boyle 2008), whereas in the past, a diagnosis of dementia almost implicitly implied the absence of mental capacity (Boyle, 2010), the erosion of rationality and the need for proxy decision-making or for family members to make decisions for that person (Hulko and Stern, 2009). The dominance of the biomedical model, where 'doing to' as opposed to 'being with' (Post, 2000, p 3) has been the norm, where people living with dementia have been silenced or not listened to (Gilmour and Brannelly, 2010), and where, in the context of dementia services, paternalistic and protective practices

(Alzheimer Europe, 2011) as opposed to those of empowerment and enablement have prevailed, have also been driving forces here.

In Chapter One I referred to Kitwood's reconceptualization of dementia and his arguing for a model of care that would support 'personhood' throughout the entire illness trajectory. For Kitwood and Bredin (1992), 'personhood' was not cognitively based but rather, it was constructed in a social context. This viewpoint contrasted strongly with that of many of the earlier philosophers who, according to some (Post, 2000; Bartlett and O'Connor, 2007; Dewing, 2008; Hughes, 2014), considered rationality, cognition and consciousness to be the hallmarks of personhood. Since dementia caused impairments to these domains, dementia was considered to usurp people of their 'personhood' (Cohen and Eisdorfer, 1986). Consider for a moment the following statement noted by Hughes (2014) and published in the *Journal of Medicine and Philosophy* in the late 1980s:

> I believe that the severely demented, while of course remaining members of the human species, approach more closely the condition of animals than normal humans in their psychological capacities. In some respects the severely demented are even worse off than animals such as dogs and horses.... The dementia that destroys memory in the severely demented destroys their psychological capacities to forge links across time that establish a sense of personal identity across time. Hence, they lack personhood. (Brock, 1988, quoted in Hughes, 2014, p 69)

Kitwood's theorizing turned these earlier appallingly reductionist philosophical understandings of personhood on their head, since for Kitwood, 'personhood' was a dynamic phenomenon, continuously in a state of flux. Indeed for Kitwood (1997a), the purpose of all dementia care was to 'maintain personhood in the face of failing mental powers' (1997a, p 84). At a time when a person's sense of security was disappearing due to memory and cognitive impairment, 'personhood', it was claimed, could be reinstated and sustained by others (Kitwood and Bredin, 1992). Promoting 'personhood' could alleviate the adverse behavioural impact of dementia.

Despite Kitwood's enormous contribution to the field of dementia studies and the most helpful insights he generated, including his challenging the notion that rationality was a critical prerequisite for 'personhood' and disentangling 'personhood' from cognitive functioning and autonomy (O'Connor and Purves, 2009), his work remains underdeveloped. His characterization of 'personhood' as a ranking, conferred on the individual by others, places that person in a passive, powerless position. It ignores the important role the individual's own everyday decision-making plays in maintaining one's sense of self and self-identity (Fetherstonhaugh et al, 2013). It also reinforces the 'us and them' divisions he himself strove to avoid. What Kitwood did achieve, however, was recognition that one's 'personhood' could be enhanced or undermined by the assumptions, values and beliefs held by others.

Since Kitwood's death, others have pointed to the overwhelming preoccupation society has with people's rational cognitive capabilities and behaviour. Post (2000) argued that we live in a hyper-cognitive society that places undue emphasis on rationality and memory. This serves to alienate people when they develop dementia. He asserted that 'dementia ethics begins with an appreciation for noncognitive well-being and a willingness to engage remaining capacities and memory …' (Post, 2000, p 13). He claimed that the value of a human being cannot be reduced because of a 'mental disorder' and 'human beings are much more than sharp minds, powerful rememberers and economic successes' (2000, p 5). According to Post, '[t]oo great an emphasis placed on rationality and memory, arguably the cardinal values of modern technological societies wrongly suggests an exclusion of people with dementia from the sphere of human dignity and respect' (2000, p 4). Like Kitwood, Post contended that despite deteriorating cognitive functioning, people can still have personhood and moral worth, even if their thinking has become impaired.

Likewise, Sabat challenged the biomedical model by questioning the inherent value of mental capacity testing (assessing the individual's ability to make decisions based on a standardized validated tool). Sabat (2005) argued that such assessments can only ever capture some but not all capacities, and claimed that despite cognitive decline, human beings remain semiotic, meaning that they act intentionally, constructing their own meaning for the situations they find themselves in. Some people, despite a dementia, will continue to have intact abilities that would otherwise be hidden if our understanding of them was based purely on standard neuropsychological testing (Sabat, 2005). In critiquing clinical approaches used to assess mental capacity, Sabat contended that it can never be assumed that a person lacks 'meaning-making ability'. People's capacity can fluctuate – in certain situations they can accomplish challenges and tasks, which in other situations would be unachievable (Sabat, 2005).

Whilst Sabat's overall contribution to the field of dementia studies has been enormous, especially his analysis of excess disability (Sabat, 1994), selfhood (Sabat, 2001), and his critique of approaches used to measure 'mental capacity' (Sabat, 2005), curiously his theorizing about dementia selfhood and mental capacity was occurring in the US during the early 2000s, the same time as negotiations were underway globally for the drafting of the CRPD, and where, in the context of disability, ongoing debates were already taking place about issues relating to 'capacity' including the distinction between 'legal status' (one's entitlement to hold rights) versus 'legal agency' (one's capacity to exercise rights) (UN enable, 2005). This is yet another example of how dementia scholars and disabilities activists, although theorizing about similar issues around the same time, appeared not to have entered into dialogue with one another or collaborated on topics central to the human rights of people with a disability like dementia.

As Article 12 of the CRPD deals with the complex issue of legal capacity in the context of the lives of people with disabilities, it is said to be the beating heart of the Convention (Nilsson, 2012). The Article is considered to be both the linchpin to the achievement of all other human rights and instrumental to personhood (Flynn and Arstein-Kerslake, 2014), and this Article, along with its ramifications for people living with dementia, is briefly reviewed in the section that follows. The review is kept deliberately brief, since Chapter Seven, written by Eilionóir Flynn, a human rights lawyer and expert on the topic, provides a more extensive critique.

Equal recognition before the law

Legal capacity is fundamental to a person's freedom and is critical for the exercise of all human rights (OHCHR, 2014) since it refers to recognition that a person is a holder of rights and obligations before the law. In this context, Article 12 on legal capacity is extremely important, especially for people with a disability, their family members, health service professionals and other care staff, as it advances civil political and social rights by conferring legal rights to autonomy to that person. Stated simply, Article 12 instructs countries that have ratified the CRPD to recognize that disabled people have legal capacity on an equal basis with others, and that disability can never justify the deprivation of legal capacity. Article 12 also stipulates that in cases where people can no longer exercise their legal capacity, assistance must be provided to them, to support their decision-making. This same support must respect their rights, will and preferences.

So what exactly does Article 12 mean for a person living with dementia? It means that irrespective of cognitive decline (deterioration in memory, language, learning, judgement, insight and so on) and any accompanying deterioration in decision-making ability, every individual has a right to be both a holder and an executor of legal rights, and must be treated equally before the law. It means that the 'status approach' – a method used traditionally where it was assumed that 'because a person [had] a certain condition [dementia] he or she inevitably [lacked] capacity' (Hughes, 2014, p 93) and where substitute decision-makers were appointed (Quinn, 2010) – is discriminatory (Shakespeare et al, 2017) must be abolished and is no longer permissible in international law (Flynn and Arnstein-Kerslake, 2014). This also means 'recognizing which decisions the person can make and which they cannot make' (Alzheimer Europe, 2016, p 58).

Based on this Article, many Western countries have outdated laws that are not in compliance with Article 12 (EU FRA, 2013b), and although some European countries have reformed their legislation to conform with Article 12, others are still operating outdated systems that continue to disempower vulnerable people, including those living with dementia (Alzheimer Europe, 2016). In this context, Ireland provides a useful example of a country that has, since December 2015, passed new and forward-thinking mental health legislation (Assisted Decision-Making [Capacity] Act 2015). This new legislation aims to promote individual autonomy and protect those whose decision-making abilities may be threatened. In effect, the new Act in Ireland is said to represent a shift in the health and social care system, since the 'functional approach' rather than the 'status approach' to capacity is evident. The functional approach views capacity not as a binary concept (no capacity or full capacity) but instead, capacity is decision-specific (Nuffield Council on Bioethics, 2009). It assesses capacity on the basis of one's ability to 'understand, recall and weigh up relevant information (as well as being able to communicate a decision)' (Hughes, 2014, p 94). The functional approach recognizes that capacity can fluctuate, and various factors (environmental and personal) will impact on decision-making ability (Alzheimer Europe, 2016). Despite the passing of this empowering legislation, at the time of writing Ireland still has not fully implemented this new legislation, and continues to operate under an antiquated system (Lunacy Regulation [Ireland] Act 1871), which denies people their human rights including their right to legal capacity. In fact, Ireland is also the only European country that to date has not ratified the CRPD.

Article 12 on legal capacity has profound implications for those living with dementia insofar as it promotes autonomy and self-determination by acknowledging a far less restrictive view of capacity. The Article is said to open up zones of freedom previously unavailable to the individual with a disability (Quinn, 2010). Building on Article 12, that all people have legal capacity and equal rights before the law, this chapter now progresses to a critical review of the individual's right to an early diagnosis, its ethical disclosure, post-diagnostic services including rehabilitation/reablement services based on a multidisciplinary assessment, and to community supports thereby enabling people the right to live at home.

The right to an early diagnosis and its disclosure

Diagnosis as a human rights issue

Article 25 (health), which recognizes that people with a disability have the right to enjoy '... the highest attainable standard of health without discrimination on the basis of disability', also asserts that States Parties shall, '[p]rovide those health services ... including *early identification and intervention* as appropriate...' (Article 25b, p 18; emphasis added). For the purpose of this book, 'early identification' is interpreted as 'early diagnosis'[1] and the section that follows examines the issue of the individual's right to an early diagnosis and their right to its ethical disclosure.

The *World Alzheimer report* (ADI, 2011) has noted that from the 1990s onwards, recognition had emerged that people had a 'right' to obtain a diagnosis and have this disclosed to them. Early diagnosis has been identified as the key to accessing dementia services (Knapp et al, 2007; Robinson et al, 2015), the gateway to medical treatments (Iliffe et al, 2009) – it is said to delay nursing home admission (Mittelman et al, 1996) and is supported by both clinical guidelines (Foley and Swanwick, 2014) and national dementia strategies (ADI, 2011; Banerjee, 2013; Fortinsky and Downs, 2014; Robinson et al, 2015). In fact, 'diagnosis along with treatment and care' are one of the seven key targets set out in WHO's recent global plan of action on dementia (WHO, 2016).

Benefits of an early diagnosis from a human rights perspective

Most types of dementia result in a progressive and irreversible decline in cognitive abilities (Alzheimer Europe, 2016) and in the individual's capacity to function independently (Nuffield Council on Bioethics,

2009). However, in the early stages many people can still make decisions about their personal welfare, exercise choice over future care options and nominate who they would want to support them in important decision-making as their condition deteriorates (Hughes, 2014). Therefore, from a human rights perspective, an early diagnosis can promote dignity and autonomy by empowering the individual to take ownership of their illness (Gilliard et al, 2005) and engage in forward planning at a time when their capacity remains intact. For example, a person can still generally, at an early stage, participate in important decision-making about drug treatments and other psychological and psychosocial interventions and service options (Nuffield Council on Bioethics, 2009).

Medical interventions, specifically cholinesterase inhibitors (drugs used for symptomatic treatment), and non-medical approaches such as counselling, and rehabilitation, are said to have maximum impact during the early stages of the course of the illness (Bamford et al, 2004; Milne, 2010). Advanced healthcare directives (statements made about future decision-making on medical treatments and healthcare) and enduring powers of attorney (nominating a trusted person to act on one's behalf regarding complex decision-making) provide excellent opportunities for the individual to exercise their rights to autonomy (Alzheimer Europe, 2016), but these protections can only be drawn up legally when the individual still has insight and capacity (Milne, 2010). It is for all these reasons that from a human rights-based perspective, an early diagnosis is so important. The diagnosis can promote and protect dignity and wellbeing (UNECE, 2015b), and enable the individual to exercise choice and control over future lifetime options. Often the person also wants to know their diagnosis, '… because giving a name to what is happening to them (or to their loved ones) is very helpful. It immediately provides a framework for understanding' (Hughes, 2014, p 47) or, as the late Sir Terry Pratchett (quoted in Alzheimer's Society, 2008, p x) wrote, 'if we are to kill the demon then first we have to say its name.' So if early diagnosis is a human right (ADI, 2011), how likely is it that the person experiencing the symptoms will receive an early diagnosis and if not, why not – what are some of the barriers to diagnosis?

Likelihood of receiving an early diagnosis

Despite the supposed benefits[2] likely to accrue to the individual and their family as a result of an early diagnosis, it is estimated that less than half of all people living with dementia in high-income countries are ever diagnosed: in low to middle-income countries the figure drops to as few as 10 per cent (Prince, 2015). Banerjee (2015) argues that this 'diagnostic gap', the number of people who should be diagnosed but are not, and the consequent 'treatment gap', the number of people with dementia who need treatment but do not get it, is even greater in low- to middle-income countries. In India, for example, he claims that about 90 per cent of cases of dementia remain unidentified. If dementia were curable, individuals would be a lot more vociferous about having their human rights fulfilled.

Across Europe, the Alcove study (Brooker et al, 2014), which examined *timely diagnosis* in 24 European countries,[3] one-quarter of which already had national dementia strategies/plans, found that between 40 to 60 per cent of cases of dementia were still being missed. Some countries fared better by missing only 30 per cent, but others fared worse and missed over 60 per cent (Brooker et al, 2014). These findings are surprising given recent policy drives, the benefits likely to accrue from an early diagnosis (Milne, 2010; ADI, 2011; Cahill and Pierce, 2013; Brooker et al, 2014) and the evidence that most people experiencing the symptoms would like to know their diagnosis (Boustani et al, 2006; Raeymaekers and Rogers, 2010; Robinson et al, 2015). Accordingly, if early diagnosis is a human right and can be beneficial to the individual and family members, why is it acceptable that the majority of people living with the syndrome remain undiagnosed and untreated (Banerjee, 2013), and what are the barriers to diagnosis?

Barriers to a timely/early diagnosis

Attitudinal

A growing body of literature demonstrates the attitudinal and structural barriers that prevent early diagnosis (see Boïse et al, 1999; Connell et al, 2004; Ilife and Manthorpe, 2004; Ilife and Wilcock, 2005; Koch and Ilife, 2010). Stigma, defined as a discrediting attribute which relegates someone from a 'whole and usual person to a tainted discounted one' (Goffman, 1963, p 12), and which can manifest in fear, shame, guilt, embarrassment and social isolation, constitutes one well-known attitudinal barrier (DH, 2009; Banerjee, 2010, 2015). Stigma, including fear of social labelling, discrimination and social exclusion, may prevent some symptomatic people from coming forward for diagnosis – the individual may resist being labelled with an illness they believe is viewed very negatively in society. Fear of multiple losses such as the loss of status, income, independence and dignity and of being demeaned, devalued and relegated to the status of a non-person, in a society that places undue emphasis on sharp minds and cognitive capabilities (Hughes, 2014), may also result in some people refraining from seeking a diagnosis. Families, too, may feel stigmatized by the illness, and may be complicit in their efforts to protect their loved one.

Some GPs can themselves have stigmatizing attitudes about dementia that prevent them from being more proactive (Iliffe et al, 2005; Vernooij-Dassen et al, 2005; Moore and Cahill, 2013; Gove et al, 2015). Some GPs may also have nihilistic views, firm in the belief that because dementia is not curable, no benefits will accrue to the individual, and hence there is no point in diagnosing or worrying the 'patient' unnecessarily. A major policy drive in virtually all national dementia strategies is to reduce stigma by developing public awareness campaigns aimed at improving understanding of dementia (Pot and Petrea, 2013).

Structural

Other barriers to obtaining an early diagnosis are structural and include the fact that diagnosing dementia for a GP is not straightforward (Robinson et al, 2015); the diagnostic work-up takes time – the first visit to a GP is said to take one hour (Wimo, 2015), and difficulties exist in differentiating dementia from normal age-related memory loss (Cahill et al, 2006). Reimbursement systems are low (Perry et al, 2011), access to diagnostic services may be difficult and challenging (Cahill et al, 2008), and a low status is often assigned to dementia services in government health and social care services (Cantley and Bowes, 2004; Banerjee, 2013). Given a consensus exists across most national dementia strategies that early diagnosis should occur in primary care (Milne, 2010; Pot and Petrea, 2013), and that GPs are as proficient as memory clinics in making the diagnosis (van Hout et al, 2000), the importance of training GPs to actively engage in diagnostic work-up and follow-up cannot be over-emphasized.

The Alcove study demonstrated that 70 per cent of countries surveyed reported that family doctors were inadequately trained to diagnose dementia (Brooker et al, 2014). In our own Irish study, where 90 per cent of GPs reported they had no dementia-specific training, 83 per cent claimed they would welcome specialist education (Cahill et al, 2006). Yet, it took another decade from the time the fieldwork for that study was undertaken before the first Irish GP reference guide for dementia was launched (Foley and Swanwick, 2014). Such time lags provide useful examples of structural discrimination as the perceived lack of time, training and support of people with dementia is probably underpinned by ageism, stereotyping and lack of value attached to older people (Gove et al, 2015).

Making dementia training a compulsory part of medical training was written down in the original Paris Declaration (Alzheimer Europe, 2006), but this has never since been explicitly articulated in countries' national dementia strategies, and whilst government plans have been very strong in their policy drive to increase diagnostic rates and provide timely interventions (ADI, 2011, 2013) (with a few countries like Scotland, Northern Ireland and England now boasting diagnostic rates of over 60 per cent) (*Scotland's national dementia strategy [2013-2016]*, see Scottish Government, 2013; *Prime Minister's challenge on dementia 2020*, see DH, 2015), targets set for the mandatory training of those responsible for diagnosis have not been clearly spelt out, nor has realistic funding been set aside for GP training. For example, whilst the upskilling of GPs in diagnosis is one of three core areas identified for investment in the Irish national dementia strategy (DoH, 2014), the funding allocated to its community awareness programme (€2.7 million) was more than double that assigned for GP training (HSE, 2016).

Disclosure as a human rights issue

Apart from having a right to a diagnosis, the individual also has a right to have the news of their diagnosis *disclosed* to them in an ethical, supportive way, respectful of their dignity, autonomy and human rights (UNECE, 2015b). Post (2000) suggests that a person should be told the truth about their diagnosis and about their prognosis and drug efficacy. Ideally, they should also be told the truth about the dementia sub-type – the exact disease causing the dementia; for example, Alzheimer's or Parkinson's disease are different types of dementia with different symptoms and different courses, and will respond differently to various treatments (Foley and Swanwick , 2014; Robinson et al, 2015). The individual should also be told the truth about alternatives to drug treatments along with the side effects and the potential risks associated with medication (Alzheimer Europe, 2016).

Disclosure should be a therapeutic rather than a horrific process (Prince, 2015), and delivered in a person-centred way (Robinson et al, 2011), with relevant information staggered over time (Iliffe and Manthorpe, 2004) rather than being delivered in a once-off encounter (Fisk et al, 2007; Iliffe et al, 2009). In other words, the right information needs to be given at the right time, in the right way; and a supportive, patient-centred approach that is realistic and fosters hope (Fisk et al, 2007) needs to be adopted during disclosure. The hazards of too much information being given at diagnosis, a time when one's information needs may be more about the 'dementia' and less about lifestyle-related matters such as driving and legal planning, were well articulated in Begley's study (2009), as the following extract illustrates:

Interviewer:	And I think that was the day that you were given your diagnosis, that's when the doctor told you what was wrong, I think.
Respondent:	Yeah, that was, that was a bit scary, you know....
Interviewer:	How did you find it?
Respondent:	Well I think he [the doctor] talked more about driving and fuckin' everything, sorry, driving, you know, get onto your thing and get, get to a solicitor and whatever that thing … see I can't remember.
Interviewer:	Enduring power of attorney.
Respondent:	Yeah, he was telling me all these things, he wasn't telling me anything about my head. (man with Alzheimer's disease, 70 years old, quoted in Begley, 2009, p 198)

Giving and receiving news of a diagnosis is an important intervention in the complex adjustment process, and where and how the news is disclosed will have far-reaching consequences for the individual and family members (Iliffe and Manthorpe, 2004; Sabat, 2005; Banerjee, 2015). A telephone call to the individual or family member (Banerjee, 2015) is an unethical and unacceptable means of conveying such critical news. Samsi and colleagues' study (2014) showed the inappropriateness of some clinical environments as the place for disclosure. Some participants in that study were highly critical of the approach taken, and disclosure was described as 'rarely a smooth process' (Samsi et al, 2014, p 8). A member of one of the working groups on dementia reported how she was first told she had mild cognitive impairment in a clinical setting. Later that same day, when returning to the car park from this appointment, where she thought she had been told her diagnosis, she bumped into the practice nurse. When she explicitly asked the nurse – had she Alzheimer's disease? – this was confirmed to her in the car park. Misinformation and the use of euphemisms may cause further confusion and yield more harm than good.

Disclosure practices

The empirical evidence suggests that many people are still not being told their diagnosis (Alzheimer Europe, 2014a), or if told, the quality of that disclosure can be problematic (Clare, 2003; ASI, 2011; Samsi et al, 2014). In their survey of 30 European countries, Alzheimer Europe (2014a) showed that in two-thirds of countries surveyed, the person was not routinely told their diagnosis, and whilst in most countries adequate information was given to the individual about drugs treatments, information on social supports was not systematically provided in about one-third of countries, and no information was given on financial and legal planning in half of the countries surveyed. These findings mirrored those from an earlier European study that showed that 82 per cent of people diagnosed claimed they were given no information about support services available (Georges, et al, 2008). Bamford et al's systematic review showed that non–disclosure or the communication of vague information was experienced as upsetting, confusing and difficult (Bamford et al, 2004).

For practical and ethical reasons it is difficult to capture empirically information about the actual discussions that take place behind closed doors between GPs and people with symptoms of dementia, or to comment on whether disclosure practices have increased since the advent of national dementia strategies (Steve Iliffe, personal communication, 2016). It is said that a gradual awareness of the possibility of a cognitive impairment developing may take place slowly over several GP encounters, making the point of disclosure difficult to identify (Steve Iliffe, personal communication, 2016), unless it is the point in time when a definitive diagnosis is recorded (rather than considered in conversation). Dementia registers (where GPs are required by health services to record all patients they diagnose) may increase diagnostic rates but will not necessarily improve disclosure rates.

Non-disclosure and rights not to know

Whilst policy initiatives directed towards increasing diagnostic rates are laudable, Brooker and colleagues (2014) caution practitioners about the potential danger of adopting a carte blanche policy approach to diagnosis. Like others (Iliffe and Manthorpe, 2004), they argue that the individual also has a right to have information about their diagnosis withheld from them, if they so wish, and comment, 'The drive towards early diagnosis in the absence of a recognition of the rights to choose when, where at what pace and whether to undergo assessment could result in an outcome that is not at all beneficial for the person or their family' (Brooker et al, 2014, p 687). All of this means that it is critical early on in the assessment process for clinicians to ascertain people's wishes regarding whether or not they would like to know their diagnosis and with whom they would like this information shared (Pinner and Bouman, 2003; Fisk et al, 2007). As mentioned earlier, with some few exceptions, most people will want to know their diagnosis (Dautzenberg et al, 2003; Pinner and Bouman, 2003; Samsi et al, 2014).

The way forward

A number of complex reasons, some attitudinal and others structural, explain why dementia continues to remain under-detected and undiagnosed in most countries across the world. Although evidence from systematic reviews reveals that training alone is insufficient to change behaviour (Perry et al, 2011), and multipronged approaches including better reimbursement systems and other organizational changes are required, the absence of training constitutes one of several barriers to early/timely diagnosis and early interventions that may deny people their fundamental rights. Educational providers need to ensure that dementia training and exposure to dementia is integrated into all medical undergraduate and postgraduate post-professional education and indeed, all other health service professional curricula (Kennerley and de Waal, 2013). The next generation of dementia strategies needs to address the issue of mandatory training of all GPs in dementia diagnosis. Given the supposed 'pivotal' role GPs are expected to play in diagnosis (ADI, 2011; Milne, 2010; Gove et al, 2015), the absence of adequate training in this context (Koch and Iliffe, 2010) acts as a barrier to human rights being upheld.

The right to rehabilitation based on multidisciplinary assessment

Apart from having a right to a diagnosis and to its sensitive disclosure, based on Article 26(1), people with dementia have a right to rehabilitation since the Article instructs that 'States Parties shall take effective and appropriate measures ... to enable persons with disabilities to attain and maintain maximum independence ... and extend comprehensive habilitation and rehabilitation services and programmes particularly in the areas of health, employment education and social services ... (p 19). Based on Article 26(a), people with dementia also have a right to a multidisciplinary assessment, since this Article states that rehabilitation should, 'Begin at the earliest possible stage and [be] based on the multidisciplinary assessment of individual needs and strengths' (p 19).

Rehabilitation and reablement

When we think about *rehabilitation*, we generally think about recovery from an accident or physical injury as, for example, postwar veterans, or the restoration of a person to their former physical health and functioning capacity, and not about recovery from dementia (Cahill and Dooley, 2005). Traditionally rehabilitation was associated with medically driven interventions delivered within a hospital setting, the goal being to achieve optimal physical functioning (Cahill and Dooley, 2005). So, given the fact that most dementias are chronic and progressive, are rehabilitation goals really achievable?

Possibly a more useful approach is to consider rehabilitation as a philosophy or a set of guiding principles (Clare, 2017) that can be used as a framework for interventions in good dementia care practice (Cohen and Eisendorfer, 1986). Here, I am guided by Marshall's (2005) early work where she identified at least four different types of rehabilitation for the individual living with dementia. According to Marshall (2005) what is common to each type is a positive approach to support and intervention. These types include rehabilitation:

- after an acute physical illness such as an infection or surgery or treatment and usually takes place in the acute care sector or in a designated rehabilitation unit;
- after a dementia-related episode of behaviours that challenge. 'These episodes often require an admission so that drug regimes can be reviewed and other interventions considered' (p 15);
- cognitive rehabilitation or making use of aspects of the brain still functioning rather than assuming nothing can be done;
- as a general approach to working in a positive way with people with dementia. 'The assumption is that most people can function better if they receive appropriate help' (p 15).

In the context of rehabilitation and dementia, I am also guided by Mishra and Barratt's (2016) more recent work where a reablement approach is introduced as part of the new narrative. This approach, they argue, challenges negative discourse since it focuses on supporting people 'to be and to do what they have reason to value' (2016, p 6). In the context of a person living with dementia, the reablement approach has application since it:

> … supports the human rights of people with dementia and their caregivers, and focuses positively on what people can do with appropriate support and interventions. It appears to actually enable people with dementia to function at their optimal capability, and offers a proactive approach that contributes to continued well-being and the prevention of crises. (Mishra and Barratt, 2016, p 18)

This more positive approach shifts the focus away from the disease model of plaques and tangles, brain atrophy, drugs and decline, to that of disability, and in keeping with the discussion forwarded in Chapter Two (see the section on the biopsychosocial model of dementia) it acknowledges 'the interplay between the intrinsic capacities of an individual and the surrounding environmental conditions' (Mishra and Barratt, 2016, p 6). The approach encourages consideration of the contextual factors (personal and environmental) likely to impact on the subjective experience of dementia including the relationships between the capacity of the individual and that person's surrounding environment (Mishra and Barratt, 2016).

It leads to further reflections on how the built and psychosocial environment can be best adapted to compensate for the individual's disability. So, rather than focusing on deficits, the emphasis is on strengths, retained abilities, what people can still do safely and what is important to them. The reablement approach encourages a person to 'gain or restore autonomy in their own space' (Mishra and Barratt, p 4), empowering them to live well and participate in everyday life at home and within their own community in a way that is meaningful to them (Clare, 2017). Within the philosophy of reablement, a variety of interventions that focus on enabling optimal functioning can then be introduced.

If we were to interpret rehabilitation to reflect this broad philosophy of reablement, that is, supporting people to function optimally in the context of their current health and ability and helping to reduce excess disability, then it could be argued that most national dementia strategies perform well in this context, although reablement tends to be done better in some countries compared with others, for example, in England, where dementia advisers and peer support networks have been made available in 40 consortium areas, and where this new service initiative has been positively evaluated (Clarke et al, 2013) and is now available across England and Scotland (personal communication with Charlotte Clarke, 2017); in Scotland where, since April 2013, a link worker is provided for the first 12 months after diagnosis (Scottish Government, 2013); and Japan, where an initial phase intensive support team is available (Nakanishi and Nakashima, 2014).

However, if we were take a more precise approach to defining rehabilitation where ideas are drawn from cognitive and behavioural psychology, and where the focus is on cognitive rehabilitation, 'a goal oriented approach to facilitate improved management of functional disability' (Clare, 2017, p 2), where therapists work collaboratively with people and target their personal goals (Clare, 2017), then current national dementia strategies are deficient. In fact, in most countries, the individual will probably never have the opportunity to exercise their right to rehabilitation based on a multidisciplinary assessment. This is despite the fact that preliminary evidence points to the benefits of cognitive rehabilitation in terms of improved outcomes for people with early stage dementia (Clare et al, 2013; Kelly and O'Sullivan, 2015; Kim, 2015; Amieva et al, 2016), and even for those with more advanced dementia (Cooper et al, 2012).

Another example of a potentially beneficial specialized intervention, but one unlikely to be widely available in most countries, is cognitive stimulation. Clare and Woods (2004) define cognitive stimulation as an intervention which:

- 'targets cognitive and/or social function
- has a social element – usually in a group or with a family care-giver,
- includes cognitive activities, which do not primarily consist of practice on specific cognitive modalities and
- may be described as reality orientation sessions or classes.' (2004, p 385)

A key difference that distinguishes cognitive stimulation from cognitive rehabilitation is that the former is group-based and consists of structured sessions used in conjunction with a manual, whilst the latter is more individualized and tailor-made.

Cognitive stimulation therapy has been found to be more cost effective that usual care (Knapp et al, 2013), and as effective as cholinesterase inhibitors (ADI, 2011), yet, in the absence of good health and social care information systems, many individuals and their family members will not become aware of this type of treatment, nor will they have the right to access it through mainstream services. As an example, a survey undertaken by Alzheimer Europe (2014a) showed that whilst cognitive and sensory stimulation interventions were available in the majority of the 27 European countries surveyed, in about half of these countries access to this service was only available through day care or long-term residential care facilities.

Multidisciplinary assessment and rehabilitation

With reference to Article 26(a), having a disability such as dementia entitles the individual to rehabilitation/reablement based on a full multidisciplinary assessment: an approach that requires input from a number of different health service professionals. The complexities associated with dementia, including cognitive, behavioural, functional, physical and emotional challenges, mean that no single speciality has the expertise to deal with these issues, and the best approach for support requires input from multiple sources (Grand et al, 2011). These include the public health nurse who may act as gatekeeper to other services, the physiotherapist who aims to increase the individual's physical mobility and independence, the occupational therapist who assesses for suitability for assistive technology and focuses on restoring and maximising the individual's independence with activities of daily living such as dressing, eating and grooming, the social worker who provides advice on service entitlement and rights and the speech and language therapist who aims to improve the individual's communication ability and cognitive function (Foley and Swanwick, 2014). Ideally what should ensue after a multidisciplinary assessment is a clear, integrated care plan detailing how the person and family member will be supported and what interventions are needed. But how likely is it that the individual's right to obtain a multidisciplinary assessment will be upheld?

The answer is that it is very unlikely, since many GPs don't have access to multidisciplinary staff (van Hout et al, 2000), and indeed, in some countries like Ireland, few fully functioning primary care teams are available (O'Riordan, 2011). Even within memory clinics (specialist centres for memory and cognitive assessment), where a full complement of health service professionals should be available, or if not, access should be readily provided (Jones, 2013), this is not always the case. Our own study of memory clinics (Cahill et al, 2014b) showed how the employment of health service professionals was patchy and inconsistent, and across Ireland only one clinic employed a full-time social worker. Where neuro-psychologists are employed in memory clinics, their focus tends to be on administering and interpreting the results of quantitative psychometric testing to support diagnostic work-up and sub-typing, and not on rehabilitation/reablement goals. Many will not have the dedicated time to focus on bespoke interventions applied to everyday living situations.

Integrally related to this discussion on early rehabilitation based on a multidisciplinary assessment is the issue of assessment for assistive technologies (AT) and for its timely installation and monitoring at home. Defined as 'Any item, piece of equipment or product system whether acquired commercially off the shelf, modified or customized that is used to increase, maintain or improve functional capabilities of individual with disabilities' (Cook and Polgar, 2013, p 5), AT has the potential to promote autonomy, independent living and improve quality of life (Cahill et al, 2004; Hagen et al, 2004). Yet the evidence suggests that it tends to be under-utilized (Mattke et al, 2011), or if used, devices are sometimes dropped into people's lives at crisis junctures, with limited information or advice made available through formal service providers on its appropriate use (Gibson et al, 2015). Whilst in the main AT could, if used ethically and appropriately, benefit the individual, from a human rights perspective, it can restrict liberty, and infringe on other human rights including the right to privacy, dignity and choice. This topic of the ethics of the use of technology is discussed in depth in Chapter Five of this book.

In reviewing a selection of national dementia strategies including the Irish (DoH, 2014), Korean (Nakanishi and Nakashima, 2014), Norwegian (Norwegian Ministry of Health and Care Services, 2015) and Luxembourg plans (Demenz, 2013), there is a notable absence of discussion within these strategies on early rehabilitation based on multidisciplinary assessment, and an absence of commitment on the part of governments to set rehabilitation targets. Where reference to multidisciplinary teams occurs, this is generally done in the context of the role community mental health teams play in *managing responsive behaviours* (Nakanishi and Nakashima, 2014), or in collecting information for clinical diagnosis (Norwegian Ministry of Health and Care Services, 2015). In the English national dementia strategy (DH, 2009), rehabilitation prospects for the individual living with dementia are only discussed in the context of hospital discharge.

Rehabilitation after surgery or acute illness

Finally, in any discussion about dementia human rights and rehabilitation/reablement, using a diagnosis of dementia as a criterion to deny the individual access to rehabilitation/reablement services following surgery or following an episode of acute illness is discriminatory and unethical. It provides another powerful example of the injustice and social exclusion some individuals will experience, especially since research evidence demonstrates that a person diagnosed with dementia can benefit significantly from specialist post-operative rehabilitation (McGilton et al, 2013). In fact, Seitz and colleagues (2016) have recently shown how post-fracture rehabilitation for older adults with dementia was associated with lower risk of long-term care admission, functional gains and lower mortality. Vassallo and colleagues (2015) have also shown how the individual diagnosed with dementia can benefit from structured rehabilitation programmes. Yet, in the same paper, the point is made that in some UK-based rehabilitation centres, people with a cognitive impairment (presumably some of whom have dementia) are explicitly excluded from these rehabilitation programmes. This may be due to nihilistic and misguided assumptions about the potential people living with a dementia have for rehabilitation, inadequate resources, the absence of staff training and other structural barriers. Although it is beyond the scope of the chapter to explore this topic in further detail, suffice to say that the area warrants more attention, especially more research and policy attention.

The right to live independently and be included in the community

In this final section of the chapter the right to live at home in the community and be supported by a range of home services is critically reviewed as are dementia-friendly communities. Article 19(a) (see Table 3.1 in Chapter Three) states that, '[p]ersons with disabilities have the opportunity to choose their place of residence and where and with whom they live on an equal basis with others and are not obliged to live in a particular living arrangement' (p 13). Article 19(b) states that '[p]ersons with disabilities have access to a range of in-home, residential and other community support services, including personal assistance necessary to support living and inclusion in the community, and to prevent isolation or segregation from the community' (p 14) (UN, 2006). A strong, positive philosophy of social inclusion and independence underpins this Article, which builds on Article 12, that all people are equal before the law, and their wishes and preferences need to be upheld.

A key policy commitment in all of the national dementia strategies reviewed for this book is to improve quality of care and support for people living with dementia at home and for their family members

(Pot and Petrea, 2013; WHO, 2016). The drive to boost community-based services is not surprising given that home care is said to offer better quality care (Moïse et al, 2004), is what most older people want (Eurobarometer, 2007; OECD, 2015), it normally costs less than institutional care (Wimo et al, 2013; Wübker et al, 2014), and people have a right to such services (UN, 2006). However, despite a rights-based ideology beginning to penetrate some countries' national strategies (see Chapters Six and Eight), with a particular emphasis on civil and political rights, social rights, including the individual's right to live at home rather than in a care home/nursing home, is nowhere explicitly spelt out, nor is any realistic funding set aside to support the provision of social care which might enable the individual to live at home indefinitely (Hughes, 2014).

The right to home care services in England

In her critique of the English national dementia strategy (DH, 2009), Boyle (2010) shows (albeit indirectly) that in England the funding assigned through the English dementia strategy (DH, 2009) to assist people to live well in the community through services such as dementia advisers (£4.5 million) and peer support networks (£3 million) has been disproportionately low compared with that assigned to the development and expansion of memory clinic assessment services (£220 million). Pointing to changes in mental health legislation that purport to offer people with dementia more autonomy, she critiques English social policy, and in particular, how the English national dementia strategy (DH, 2009) fails to offer access to social care services, support that might otherwise promote autonomy and provide realistic alternatives to institutional care. Boyle (2010) argues that the absence of government commitment to social care services, as reflected in its failure to set down targets to expand home care support, acts as a key barrier to enabling people to exercise their social rights to remain living at home.

The right to home care services in Ireland

In Ireland, government policy has, for years, been directed at ensuring that the person diagnosed with dementia is supported to live independently in the community for as long as possible (O'Shea and O'Reilly, 1999; Cahill, 2010), and like other countries, a commitment to home care is strongly embedded in the Irish national dementia strategy (DoH, 2014). However, unlike many European countries, no legislation exists in Ireland granting entitlement to social care services. In contrast, entitlement to long-term residential care exists and is based on a rigorous assessment (Nursing Home Support Scheme Act 2009). A likely outcome of this policy is that older people may be unnecessarily and prematurely admitted to nursing homes or care homes due to the paucity of community-based services and the in-built bias in government policy. Recent Irish research based on social workers' caseloads has shown that in around 50 per cent of cases, the admissions of older people, including those with dementia, to nursing homes could have been averted if appropriate home care services, including dementia-specific supervisory services, were available (Donnelly et al, 2016).

The recent allocation through the Irish national dementia strategy (DoH, 2014) of an additional €22 million to deliver intensive home care packages to people living with dementia in the community is a most welcome policy development, and serves to counter the Irish policy bias that has traditionally favoured institutional/residential care (O'Shea and Carney, 2016). However, the new allocation caters for a very small percentage (1.6 per cent) of the around 30,000 Irish people likely to be living with dementia in the community and fortunate to be residing in certain geographical areas. Whilst the Irish national dementia strategy, like the English strategy (DH, 2009) and the more recent *Prime Minister's challenge on dementia* (DH, 2015), fail to enable the individual to exercise their social rights, the new investment in home care packages in Ireland represents a shift in policy direction, in a country where dementia has traditionally been over-medicalized (O'Shea and Carney, 2016), and where home care services were in the past fragmented, inflexible and inequitably distributed (O'Shea and O'Reilly, 1999; Cahill et al, 2012; Bobersky, 2013).

The right to home care services across Europe

This absence of adequate government support to enable people with dementia to live at home in the community is not unique to England and Ireland. Across Europe, the EU RightTimePlaceCare study (Bökberg et al, 2015), which collected data on community services across the UK, France, Sweden, Spain, the Netherlands, Finland, Estonia and Germany, found a significant absence of dementia specialist services across Europe and a major gap between service provision and service utilization. Even basic services, such as home-delivered meals, home help, housing adaptations, personal safety alarms and transport services, tended to be under-utilized. In this pan-European study, specialist dementia care services considered by some to be critical to sustaining home care (Ward-Griffin et al, 2012) were seldom available, and even when they were available, they were rarely used. No two people with dementia are alike, and the heterogeneity of individuals living with dementia requires a reconfiguration of dementia services (Clarke et al, 2013) and more rights-based approaches, reflecting diversity, flexibility and equality.

On balance, and based on the evidence marshalled in this chapter, it can be concluded that choice and control over where one lives, at home or in a nursing home, is not readily available to many individuals diagnosed with more moderate to severe dementia, since mainstream social care services are often inadequate (Argyle et al, 2010; Bobersky, 2013, Bökberg et al, 2015; UNECE, 2015b) relative to long-term care (Ranci and Pavolini, 2015). Even in countries with better-developed community services, inadequate personal budgets and inadequate support for family members limits choice (Ilinca et al, 2015).

The right to home care services for people with severe dementia

Of course the issue of a person with severe dementia being free to choose where and with whom they wish to live is highly contentious and raises ethical and moral questions, given the excessive financial costs of 24-hour home care, safety concerns, the notion of proportionality (Hughes, 2010) and the need to protect the human rights of others. Autonomy needs must be balanced alongside safety rights and risks (Robinson et al, 2007) and the rights of family members and service providers. What is at stake here, is that the individual should never be forced against their wishes to relocate to a nursing home or care home and deception and lies should not be used to coerce those with a severe dementia to leave their homes, as this type of unethical behaviour may make the adjustment process all the more difficult (Bobersky, 2013). Ideally, a range of attractive long-term care options, including housing with care, group dwellings, specialist care units, and dementia villages and nursing homes, should be available, and as far as possible, the individual's rights and preferences should be respected and balanced against the rights and wishes of other family members responsible for that person's support.

Dementia-friendly communities

Finally, in keeping with the biopsychosocial model of disability advanced in Chapter Two of this book, and the philosophy of reablement introduced earlier in this chapter, if the individual is to be helped to live an ordinary life and remain active in their local communities, then dementia, like disability, needs to be made more visible and normalized across all communities (Nuffield Council on Bioethics, 2009; WHO, 2012), and people's collective rights, including their right to be socially included, participate in meaningful activities and be treated with dignity and respect, need to be upheld.

Dementia-friendly communities have been defined as those where 'people with dementia are empowered to have high aspirations and feel confident, knowing that they can contribute and participate in activities that are meaningful to them' (Alzheimer's Society, 2013c, p viii). They are a good example of the disability/social model at play (McGettrick, 2014), since the approach reflects a shift from the biomedical model with its emphasis on clinical assessments, physical health and cognitive functioning to a more holistic social model, supporting people to enjoy a good quality of life within their own communities (Rees, 2015). Much has been written about this particular social movement (see, for example, ADI, 2015b; Alzheimer Europe, 2015; UNECE 2015b; Wiersma and Denton, 2016), since the concept first gained traction in Japan over 10 years ago (Rees, 2015; Bartlett, 2016).

However, in terms of human rights, what exactly do dementia-friendly communities mean, especially to the experts, people living with dementia? Swaffer (2014) asserts that whilst the approach is well-aligned with the disability model of dementia and with a human rights framework, dementia-friendly communities may recreate inequalities if agenda-setting is done by others, and if people living with dementia are not seen as equal partners. Bartlett (2016), an academic, in applying a social citizenship lens to her analysis, and drawing on the English experience (where energy for such initiatives first emerged from the government and the Alzheimer's Society, and not from non-state actors), questions the respective roles of state and non-state actors in determining people's citizenship rights and the power struggles that may emerge if ordinary citizens are not involved as equal partners in these initiatives. Others (see Shakespeare et al, 2017, p 6) claim that *dementia-friendly communities* and *dementia friends* reflect a weak social response to dementia. They believe what is most needed is 'an equalities-based approach' that demands entitlements.

My own critique is that whilst undoubtedly the dementia-friendly community agenda holds promise, in terms of building social capital, combating social exclusion and creating links that may in the future foster trust and solidarity, for dementia-friendly communities to be effective and sustainable, they will need to be adequately resourced.

And whilst dementia-friendly communities are about human rights (Rees, 2015), and in particular, civil and political rights, how exactly can the agenda advance economic rights? There is also the risk that the dementia-friendly movement will become 'all things to all people' (Bulmer, 2015, p 214): to the politician, a vote catcher; to the retailer, a new consumer group; to the service provider, a reduced caseload; and to the individual, the prospects of being labelled and having all their behaviour seen only through the dementia. Of real concern is the fact that governments and policy-makers may consider dementia-friendly communities low-cost solutions (Imogen Blood and Associates, 2017) to the heightening challenge that dementia poses.

Conclusion

This chapter has critically reviewed a selection of human rights that are often denied of community-dwelling people living with dementia and their family members. The discussion showed that despite significant policy drives to increase diagnostic rates, and improve treatments and other therapeutic outcomes, dementia still remains under-diagnosed, and is particularly invisible in low- to middle-income countries. This means that most people's right to obtain treatments, access psychosocial interventions and engage in advanced care planning will not be respected. Whilst the reasons for this are complex, structural barriers, including in the case of GPs, their lack of time, lack of training, poor access to the necessary specialist and diagnostic services, therapeutic nihilism and ageism, are likely contributors.

Educational providers need to integrate dementia training into all health service professional training and all medical, nursing and health science undergraduate and postgraduate education (Kennerley and de Waal, 2013). The accreditation of all nursing, medical, psychology and allied health courses should be contingent on the inclusion of dementia as a priority topic. The next generation of national dementia strategies must address the issue of the mandatory training of GPs in dementia diagnosis and its ethical and timely disclosure. Training should be based on research, and should ideally involve people living with dementia.

The discussion also showed that in line with the CRPD, the individual living with dementia has a right to early rehabilitation based on a multidisciplinary assessment and to live at home in the community with adequate home care supports. It showed that whilst policy plans generated by many countries today are committed to the broad principles and philosophy of reablement, a biopsychosocial approach, which provides a broader framework for interventions

(Spector et al, 2016), and takes cognizance of the wide range of factors likely to impact on the individual's experience including biological, psychological, cultural, familial and socioeconomic (O'Shea and Carney, 2016), is not in evidence in most countries. This chapter also critically reviewed the individual's right to choose to live at home and have access to a range of in-home care supports. It was argued that a lack of commitment on the part of most governments to provide realistic home care supports results in some people being prematurely admitted to long-stay residential care.

The way forward is one that recognizes the importance of reframing dementia in social terms, to improve the individual's quality of life, just like what the social model of disability achieved for people with a disability (O'Shea and Carney, 2016). The optimum model is one that takes a whole-person biopsychosocial approach, gives power and control back to the individual and their family members, and allows for recognition of the individual's rights. The CRPD, especially Articles 12 and 19, provide opportunities for the equal participation of people with dementia in society and for their inclusions in the all-important aspects of decision-making. The chapter that follows shifts the focus away from care and support at home in the community to review a range of other human rights critically important to those living with dementia in long-stay residential care.

Summary of key points

- Article 12 recognizes that a person with a disability has legal capacity and is the holder of rights and obligations before the law.
- Article 12 therefore has important implications for a person living with dementia as it promotes the individual's autonomy rights, considers capacity to be decision-specific and rules out disempowering approaches which, in the past, were used to assess capacity.
- Governments and policy-makers need to ensure that all policies, legislation and guidelines relating to dementia comply with Article 12.
- Obtaining a diagnosis of dementia is a human right but conversely, refraining from obtaining a diagnosis is also a human right.
- An early diagnosis can promote dignity and wellbeing, maximize autonomy and enable the individual to exercise choice and control over future lifetime options.
- Globally, dementia diagnostic rates remain very low, and because of this, most people are denied the opportunity to obtain treatments and gain access to other non-pharmacological interventions likely to promote their quality of life.
- A complex range of attitudinal and structural barriers prevent many people from obtaining an early diagnosis.

- Training in dementia assessment diagnosis and disclosure should be made mandatory for all medical doctors.
- Dementia diagnosis and disclosure should be a supportive process where people are told the truth about the syndrome, its likely cause and what the future holds.
- A biopsychosocial approach provides a useful framework for practitioners working in the field as it allows for the consideration of biological, psychological, cultural, familial and socioeconomic factors likely to impact on the individual's experience of dementia.
- People living with dementia are entitled to a multidisciplinary assessment that provides them and their family members with an integrated care plan.
- People living with dementia should never be refused rehabilitation services.
- In keeping with Article 19, a person diagnosed with dementia is entitled to live at home in the community or in a place of their choice with personal supports.

Notes

[1]   Over the last 10 years it has been argued that the term 'timely diagnosis' may be more person-centred and therefore more preferable to the term 'early diagnosis' (Alzheimer Europe, 2014a). A core difficulty here is that several different interpretations of the term 'timely diagnosis' now exist, ranging from 'the time when the patient or caregiver and the primary care physician first recognize that a dementia syndrome may be developing' (de Lepeleire et al, 2008) to the right time for the particular patient and doctor in their particular circumstances (Dhedhi et al, 2014) to a time when benefits of diagnosis are balanced against risks (Nuffield Council on Bioethics, 2009). It is for this reason that in this chapter I adhere to the expression 'early diagnosis', which is that originally used by the European Parliament in their written declaration and in their fight against Alzheimer's disease (Grossetete et al, 2008).

[2]   It should be remembered that these benefits are more conjectural than evidence-based (ADI, 2011).

[3]   The Alcove study also investigated other aspects of dementia besides merely timely diagnosis.

FIVE

The right to a good quality of life in care homes or in nursing homes

> The elderly individual wandering the street is easily identified as homeless yet there is an entire population of elders who suffer silently enduring the painful state of homelessness within the confines of the total institution of the nursing home. (Carboni, 1990, p 37)

Introduction

In this chapter the focus shifts from care at home to support in a nursing home or care home where many older people who have a more moderate to severe dementia live. There is evidence to suggest that people with dementia are over-represented amongst nursing home and care home residents (ADI, 2013). For example over two thirds of people living in care homes or nursing homes in Ireland, the US and England probably have dementia (Cahill et al, 2010; Alzheimer's Association, 2012; Prince et al 2014).

According to the ADI (2013), care homes[1] for people living with dementia typically consist of, 'residential care, or assisted living facilities staffed by care assistants … nursing homes, staffed by registered nurses as well as nursing and care assistants … [and] dementia special care units [SCUs] staffed by specialist dementia nurses, and attended by multidisciplinary care teams … for those with advanced dementia…' (ADI, 2013, p 33). Despite policy drives over the last two decades in some European countries, especially the Netherlands (Verbeek, 2013), to increase the provision of SCUs, most people in Europe and in the US who need long-term care because of dementia live in residential homes or care homes (Alzheimer Europe, 2013; Harris-Kojetin et al, 2013; Cahill et al, 2015a).

A care home is a person's home, their permanent place of residence for an indefinite period of time. How, with whom, and where the individual spends their time and the quality of their interactions there (Harmer and Orrell, 2008; Theurer et al, 2015) will significantly impact on quality of life (Moyle et al, 2015; Jing et al, 2016). Building on the work of Kitwood (1997a), who located 'behaviours that challenge' not in the brain but in the individual's emotional ill-being, it is argued that despite policy plans that purport to promote quality in residential care (ADI, 2013), the biomedical model for contextualizing dementia prevails, and some individuals living with dementia in care homes are being exposed to suboptimal and at the extreme, harmful practices, and to regimes of control and restriction (Alzheimer Europe, 2012). Such practices violate human rights including the right to be treated equally, to dignity, privacy, independence and autonomy. We can do a lot more to improve the quality of life and quality of care for people with moderate to severe dementia living in long-term residential care.

Against the backdrop of key concepts introduced in earlier chapters including personhood, excess disability, participation and autonomy, this chapter critically reviews the following four Articles enshrined in the CRPD, namely, the right to:

- protection from torture or cruel, inhuman or degrading treatment or punishment
- accessibility and especially access to the physical environment
- respect for privacy
- participate in cultural life, recreation and leisure.

At the outset it must be remembered that each of these rights straddle other Articles contained in the CRPD, but in the interest of space, it is impossible to review all 50 Articles. Therefore, by operationalizing a limited selection of Articles, this chapter provides a fresh conceptual lens to explore the everyday subjective experiences of some individuals living with dementia in care homes. Drawing on the relevant empirical research, and comparing the evidence against provisions set out in the Articles, the aim is to make a link between practical actions and human rights. Recommendations are forwarded about how autonomy, dignity, independence and privacy rights can be enhanced, and how decision-making, choice and control can be returned to the individual.

Townsend (2006) reminds us of the scale of human rights violations and the level at which rights can be fulfilled; this chapter concentrates on what constitute more insidious rights, relevant to people *already* resident in care homes. It must be remembered that irrespective of the scale of violation, any human rights breach can be serious (Townsend, 2006, Kelly and Innes, 2012) as it can undermine the very core of the individual's humanity, personhood and agency, and can result in lasting psychological harm (Sabat, 2005). The abuse of human rights can also challenge the essence of what Kitwood (1997a) characterizes as person-centred care, since the individual's integrity can be slighted and the person stripped of dignity and self-worth (Kelly and Innes, 2012).

At the outset, it is also important to create a realistic picture of some of the moral and ethical dilemmas health service professionals and care staff encounter when supporting the complex needs of the individual living with dementia, especially when care homes are not purpose-built, when some frontline care staff have had no opportunities for training, and feel overworked (Brooker and Latham, 2016), poorly paid (WHO, 2012; OECD, 2015) and may be unsupported. Providing 'quality care' is resource-intensive and carries significant financial costs (Wübker et al, 2014), and many front-line care staff work in conditions that are far from ideal, and have exceptionally heavy and stressful workloads. Balancing risk and safety needs against the individual's right to autonomy and independence is one key dilemma that is often encountered (Robinson et al, 2007), as is 'proportionality' and the need to take cognizance of the rights of others including residents who are cognitively intact but physically frail. Responding to 'behaviours that challenge' such as agitation and aggression (Konetzka et al, 2014) or 'intrusive behaviour' and 'wandering' (Maunder, 2013) by locking some individuals in units, essentially warehousing the person (Kitwood, 1997a) and controlling such behaviours with physical and chemical restraints, may exacerbate behaviours and violate human rights.

Article 15(1) and 15(2) of the CRPD (UN, 2006, p 12) states that, 'no one shall be subjected to torture or to cruel, inhuman or degrading treatment or punishment', and that, 'States Parties shall take all effective legislative, administrative judicial or other measures to prevent persons with disabilities, on an equal basis with others, from being subjected to ... [such treatments or punishment].' In this chapter, I use the ECHR's definition of 'degrading treatment', which conceptualizes it as, 'treatment or punishment that arouses in the victim a feeling of fear, anguish and inferiority capable of humiliating and debasing them' (Kelly, 2005, p 11).

In the section that follows, the right to protection from such treatment is discussed against the backdrop of the use of chemical and physical restraints and assistive/surveillance technology. The second part of the chapter advances to an exploration of accessibility rights especially rights to access the physical environment. The third part deals with privacy rights and the final part concludes with an exploration of the individual's rights to remain socially engaged and to participate in meaningful activities, in a care home and outside.

Freedom from torture or cruel, inhuman or degrading treatment or punishment

Residential care settings are the homes of many older people who, despite their frailty and health problems (including dementia), should be supported to enjoy a good quality of life, maintain and develop relationships and contribute to society (ADI, 2013). Whilst ambulant, the individual should be encouraged to mobilize in a safe, stimulating and supportive environment (Post, 2000; Alzheimer Europe, 2012), and whether ambulant or not, they should be supported to access outdoor areas (Welsh et al, 2003), remain autonomous (Murphy and Welford, 2012) and engage in activities that are meaningful to them (Theurer et al, 2015). Autonomy, choice, control and participation in decision-making are critical components of quality of life for people living in care homes (Murphy and Welford, 2012). They are also key standards of care that are not always met in residential care settings (ADI, 2013).

Life in long-stay care occurs behind closed doors, often at a distance from people's own communities, and in environments that are generally not open for public scrutiny (Meenan et al, 2016). The complexities of dementia and its multiple impairments, including linguistic deficits, means that the person may be unable to complain about matters critical to their health and wellbeing; indeed, even if they do, their complaints may not always be taken seriously. Ironically, despite the strengthening of user rights and the alleged reduction in the power of health service professionals, the risk of violating a person's rights, including their mental and physical integrity, increases with a person's vulnerability (Gjerberg et al, 2013). In other words, the more severe the dementia, the more likely it is that some individuals will receive inappropriate treatment (Post, 2000; Sormunen et al, 2007). Accordingly, when no longer able to speak up for themselves (Kitwood, 1997a), there is a heightened risk of some individuals having their fundamental rights threatened or denied.

Behaviours that challenge

A person's 'behaviour' can be defined as 'challenging' if it puts them or those around them at risk or leads to a poor quality of life. Many individuals enter care homes because of these behaviours (ADI, 2013) or develop such behaviours following admission (Benoit et al, 2006; Verbeek, 2011; Bobersky, 2013). Much controversy exists regarding their exact cause, including the extent to which such behaviours are understood and responded to as symptoms of the neurodegenerative disease – a biomedical explanation and commonly referred to as the 'behavioural and psychological symptoms of dementia' (BPSD) – or alternatively, whether they reflect reactions to the social milieu, a social psychological explanation, and commonly referred to as 'behaviours that challenge', 'responsive behaviours' or 'challenging behaviours'. The reality is that a complex interplay probably exists between biological, psychological, environmental and social factors, which most likely cause the behaviours (Brooker et al, 2016).

Chemical restraints

Irrespective of cause, a consensus exists that non-pharmacological interventions, including person-centred care approaches, should always be the first line of response (Fossey et al, 2006; NICE/SCIE, 2007; Alzheimer Europe, 2012; Gjerberg et al, 2013; Brooker et al, 2016). Antipsychotic medication, also known as neuroleptics or drugs (tranquilizers), should only ever be prescribed when symptoms are severe, where there is immediate risk of harm, and when risks and benefits have been fully discussed and a comprehensive assessment undertaken (NICE/SCIE, 2007). Indeed, some believe that these drugs that were originally developed to treat psychosis and schizophrenia are never appropriate for an individual diagnosed with dementia (Alzheimer Europe, 2012).

Studies have shown the very harmful effects of antipsychotic medication when prescribed to some people who have dementia, including excess mortality, stroke and gait disturbances (Banerjee, 2009; Harding and Peel, 2013; Coon et al, 2014; Kales et al, 2015). Banerjee's review and estimates (2009) suggested how antipsychotic drugs accounted for approximately 1,800 cases of excess mortality in the UK per year and about 1,600 cases per year of cerebrovascular accidents or strokes. He claimed that these drugs were probably only effective in about one-fifth of cases.

Other studies have shown the adverse effects these drugs have on quality of life (Black et al, 2012; Clare et al, 2014). Narratives are powerful in bringing alive social phenomena, and Banerjee's review (2009), where he appealed for their more cautious use in care homes in England, drew on caregiver and service providers' accounts to contextualize experiences and to demonstrate their at times adverse effects. Consider the following comment made by a family member who was cited in Banerjee's report:

> I hold them [antipsychotics] responsible for his rapid loss of speech, the constant drooling, his mask-like frozen expression, the constant jerking of his right foot that stayed with him for the rest of his life, and rapid onset of incontinence. While still able to walk, he would walk leaning over sideways or backwards at an alarming angle and no doubt it was this unbalancing that caused the hip fracture. Soon he developed epileptic fits and I cannot be sure that it was not related to the antipsychotics. (Family carer of a person with dementia now living in a care home, quoted in Banerjee, 2009, p 16)

The rich narrative here reflects the cascade of health problems including aphasia (loss of ability to produce language), apathy, incontinence, tremors, mobility and epilepsy that this family member believed the antipsychotic drugs may have caused. Banerjee's appeal (2009) was not new, since as early as 2004 the European Medicines Agency issued a public warning about the increased risk of cerebrovascular adverse events (strokes) and mortality in elderly people with dementia being prescribed certain antipsychotic drugs (EMA, 2008).

The avoidance of, or at the very least, very cautious use of, antipsychotic medication is also a strong policy directive embedded in several countries' recent and past dementia strategies (see, for example, DH, 2009, 2015; Scottish Government, 2013; DoH, 2014; Australian Government Department of Health, 2015; ASPE, 2016).

Yet despite policy objectives, government warnings and empirical research findings, prescription rates of antipsychotic medication remain high (Engedal, 2005; Schneider et al, 2006; de Siún et al, 2014; Coon et al, 2014; Konetzka et al, 2014), and the biomedical model or technical approach to understanding and responding to dementia prevails. This is despite the fact that a burgeoning body of research exists pointing to the beneficial effects of non-pharmacological approaches for addressing 'behaviours that challenge' (Magai et al, 2002; Fossey et al, 2006; Spector et al, 2013; Zimmerman et al, 2013; Brooker et al, 2016). Indeed, a recent study of 12 Western European countries (Janus et al, 2016) demonstrated that despite warnings about side effects and recommendations for the use of non-pharmacological interventions, antipsychotic use in nursing homes ranged from 12 to 59 per cent. In selected studies focusing only on people living with dementia, the highest rates of antipsychotic drug use were found in Spain, Austria and Germany and the lowest in Norway (Janus et al, 2016). In another study (Szczepura et al, 2016) that investigated the association between England's *Living well with dementia: A national dementia strategy* (DH, 2009), (where guidelines on the cautious use of antipsychotic medication in care homes were set out) and new recommendations forwarded, no reduction in antipsychotic drug use was seen. In this same study, the length of time residents remained on treatment was also found to be excessive.

Returning to Article 15 of the CRPD, it could be argued that except in rare cases, where short-term, modest, beneficial effects may occur (Ballard et al, 2009), the inappropriate and excessive prescription of antipsychotic medication to the individual diagnosed with dementia constitutes cruel, inhuman and degrading treatment, and is a violation of human rights. If used when no attempt is made to trial other social psychological and environmental approaches, this treatment can also violate other human rights, including the right to respect for physical and mental integrity (Article 17) and to liberty and security (Article 14). Indeed, this type of treatment could verge on 'objectification' – the person is seen as a body to be controlled and technically measured rather than an individual with whom social and relational interaction is so critical (Kitwood, 1997a). If similar drugs with such poor outcomes were prescribed to children with Down's syndrome or teenagers with anorexia nervosa and not to older, frail, mostly women living with dementia, public outcry would no doubt be enormous.

So why is it acceptable that this pattern of drug prescription remains so prevalent? Why do some countries fare better than others in relation to prescription rates? Why is antipsychotic use more prevalent in more deprived geographical areas (Szczepura et al, 2016)? The answers to these questions are complex, and the reasons I suspect are multiple. At a macro level, they include the power of pharmaceutical companies, the dominance of the biomedical model, the inflexibility of sociopolitical systems, the absence of public and professional awareness about the potentially harmful effects of antipsychotic drugs, the absence of staff training and the unwillingness of advocacy groups to challenge government policies including health reimbursement systems that favour drug treatments over social, psychological and environmental interventions.

As an example, in Ireland, a nursing home, at no extra cost to the individual who generally has a medical card (a card that entitles access to GPs, other health service professionals and benefits free of charge), can request a GP or old age psychiatrist to assess a resident who exhibits 'behaviours that challenge'. Following assessment and in the absence of non-pharmacological interventions, the medical doctor may prescribe antipsychotic medication. However, if that same facility employs a therapist to provide an intervention such as, for example, cognitive stimulation therapy, significant out-of-pocket costs will result.

Care facilities with good staff-to-resident ratios tend to have a reduced rate of antipsychotic use for residents with 'behaviours that challenge' (Konetzka et al, 2014). Likewise, segregated care or purpose-built small-scale environments are associated with a better quality of life and reduced antipsychotic use (Weyerer et al, 2010). These approaches, however, are resource-intensive and carry significant financial costs. For these reasons it is likely that drugs will be used not so much for the genuine relief of symptoms, but as a labour saving and cost-controlling mechanism (Kitwood, 1997a) in care homes.

Physical restraints

Whilst chemical restraints, if used inappropriately, can contravene human rights and at the extreme, lead to untimely deaths (Banerjee, 2009), physical restraints can also, depending on their use, violate the individual's civil and political rights by subjecting a person to cruel, inhuman and degrading treatment. Physical restraints refer to devices attached to or near a person's body that deliberately prevent that person from moving about independently (Retsas, 1998). Defining what constitutes a physical restraint is not straightforward, however, as many different devices can be used. Alzheimer Europe (2012) provide examples that include '... straps and belts, strait-jackets, limb holders or mittens and in certain circumstances various medical devices such as tubes and drips', and claims that physical restraints can include 'bed rails, bed nets, or cages, trays fixed to chairs, wheelchair brakes and bars' (Alzheimer Europe, 2012, p 47). Safety concerns, risk avoidance or the control/reduction of agitation are key reasons forwarded to justify the use of restraints in long-term residential care (Capezuti, 2004; Wang and Moyle, 2005), yet the research evidence demonstrates that restraint use is not good practice, and actually yields no significant benefit (Tilly and Reed, 2006; Konetzka et al, 2014).

Interestingly, despite legislation, guidelines and policies out-ruling or at the very least significantly restricting their use, physical restraints are regularly used in care homes, and in dementia care (Hamers et al, 2004; Alzheimer Europe, 2012). A recent study (Foebel et al, 2016) showed that physical restraint use was associated with a higher risk of both functional and cognitive decline compared with chemical restraint, and risks to the individual were even more excessive when both forms of restraints were used simultaneously. In an Australian study, Peisah and Skladzien, (2014) estimated the prevalence of physical restraint use to be between 12 to 49 per cent, and earlier studies (see Kirkevold and Engedal, 2004; Hamers and Huizing, 2005) estimated similar and in some cases even higher usage.

Much of the published research on physical restraints and dementia fails to contextualize dementia as a disability, and fails to address the important issue of 'excess disability' (see Chapter Four for a definition) that physical restraints may cause. Nor, with few exceptions (see Kelly, 2010), is there much coverage in the dementia care literature on how the individual may react to the use of such restraints. Accordingly, whilst the clinical side effects of physical restraint use including ulcers, reduced muscle strength and increased dependence and agitation are well documented (Castle, 2006), far less is known about the long-term, emotional, social and psychological harm physical restraints can cause.

A further complication is that physical restraints may assault personhood and violate human rights but first person accounts of these incidents are rare. Some years ago, as part of a study on quality of life and dementia in residential care (Cahill and Diaz-Ponce, 2011), I interviewed an 80-year-old man who had a severe vascular dementia (MMSE was 4), and who was strapped into a wheelchair. The interview schedule used to collect data on quality of life contained 15 simple questions, examples of which include 'What makes you happy, what makes you sad and what do you like most about living here?' In replying to these questions, this man's responses were monosyllabic, with no eye contact; in fact, to all intents and purposes, he was mute until I came to the final question on the interview schedule, which was, 'Is there anything that could be done to improve your life here [in the nursing home]?' Then suddenly the elderly man's eyes lit up and he cogently exclaimed: "Yes, get rid of the straps, the chains around you, that's about all."

Data like these provide useful insights into the type of psychological harm (Sabat, 2005), indignity and assault on personhood and on human rights (Kelly and Innes, 2012) physical restraints can cause. Yet with sole reliance on the neurological lens to understand and respond to dementia, it is easy to assume that all behaviour, mood and deterioration, in this case, that might have been interpreted as 'apathy', 'depression' and 'aphasia', is caused by the neurological impairment, and that behavioural aberrations are a symptom of brain pathology (Sabat, 2005).

This elderly man's words remind us of how the person, or 'core self', always remains inside each and everyone of us, even those living with a severe dementia (Kitwood, 1997a), and failure to hold human beings in personhood and to treat them as commodities is synonymous with cutting them off from important relationships, which contribute so significantly to their humanity (Lindemann, 2014). This man lived in a care home where, based on my own observations (I had spent several weeks there as part of the research study), a strong emphasis was placed not on personhood but on technical task completion and clinical body care (Doyle and Rubinstein, 2014).

Haunted by what I had heard and observed, next time I returned there, I brought with me a DVD on 'Challenging Behaviours', and gently entered into discussions with the Director of Nursing about the prospects of staff training. Returning there several weeks later, I noticed that this DVD remained in the exact same place on the mantelpiece in the Director's office. The incident reminded me of how once an old culture of care becomes embedded (Doyle and Rubinstein, 2013) it is usually very difficult to change (Kitwood, 1997a; O'Shea and Carney, 2016). Good leadership in dementia care and staff training, including training on how to deliver person-centred care (Brooker, 2004) and on human rights (Kelly and Innes, 2012), is vital to the wellbeing of the individual diagnosed with dementia. Conversely, the absence of training leaves older people diagnosed with dementia extremely vulnerable and at risk of neglect and at the extreme, abusive practices (OECD, 2015; UNECE, 2015b).

While it is highly unlikely that a person with a severe dementia will complain to staff about practices or policies that threaten their human rights, family members may also feel silenced, fearful of reporting their concerns in case of recrimination (Happell, 2005). In another study (Bobersky, 2013) a poignant account was given, this time from the perspective of a family member, of a lady who was physically tied to a chair, in a care home, because she was allegedly "walking a lot". Her elderly husband who had first supported her at home for as long as he could, said:

> [My wife did] this [makes a gesture of snipping scissors], kind of "cut the restraints" all day [trying to cut the belt tying her to the chair]. It was heart-breaking [sighs]. I should not have let it happen.... But you see, what was going to happen was *if we had complained they would have told us "take her home"*. But that's something we couldn't, something we just couldn't, no, we couldn't take her home. And then we couldn't get her anywhere else in. So we had to put up with it. (Elderly Husband caregiver, quoted in Bobersky, 2013, p 158; emphasis added)

The narrative here reflects how easily a person's normal behaviour, *walking about*, can become pathologised, and then every aspect of the person is seen through the 'disease' (Sabat, 2014). The 'person' becomes 'the dementia', so to speak, and is then *managed* by those who hold power and who determine the type of intervention (ethical or otherwise) they believe is needed (Gjerberg et al, 2013). The asymmetry of power relations in nursing homes is also evident in the qualitative data, as is the lack of choice available in relation to alternate long-term care options.

In circumstances like these, one form of redress for family members may be found in advocacy services or Ombudsman services. Knowledge of mental health legislation, human rights legislation, along with an awareness of the principles and Articles enshrined in the CRPD, may also empower relatives to question practices that violate human rights. Alzheimer Europe (2012) has argued that there is a lack of rigorous legislation, recommendations and guidelines in place in relation to the use of physical restraints in dementia care.

But, it is also important to create a balanced account of the reality of everyday life for staff employed in care homes and for the residents who have dementia. When restraints are used to promote safety and enhance autonomy, and where every effort is made to gain consent or assent (where agreement to participate is given non-verbally or through behaviour) from the individual, then the situation may be reasonably straightforward (Nuffield Council on Dementia, 2009). However, where a person's decision-making ability is significantly compromised, and where physical restraints are used unethically, with no attempt made to gain the individual's consent/assent or to communicate the rationale behind their use, these interventions are illegal and unethical (Post, 2000; Alzheimer Europe, 2010). Such involuntary and inappropriate restraint use contravenes Article 15 and also breaches several of the principles set out in the CRPD, including the right to autonomy, dignity, independence, equality and choice.

A more subtle form of physical restraint often used in care homes is where internal doors are locked: areas are cordoned off and residents are forbidden from entering certain rooms, usually kitchens or staff rooms. Many years ago I spent time in an SCU, which was profit-oriented, medically driven, deficit-focused and therapeutically nihilistic (Kitwood, 1997a; Baldwin and Capstick, 2007). Here, allegedly in the interest of safety and wellbeing, all residents were locked out of their bedrooms during the day, an appalling policy that contravenes human rights legislation and which, I have been told, has since changed. In contrast, last year I spent an afternoon in a Swedish SCU in Jönköping where all internal rooms, including the staff room, were fully accessible to ambulant residents. Interestingly, although the staff room was equipped with a computer, swivel chairs and filing cabinets, it also contained a large comfortable couch, used by residents passing by, keen to stop and interact with staff at work. This SCU accommodated 10 people, all of whom had a moderate to severe dementia. Although situated on the third floor, it had an outdoor under-cover balcony, safely designed to enable residents' access to fresh air and to enjoy sensory stimulation.

My visit there was in the autumn, and I noticed a range of colourful autumnal leaves on display on a large table on the balcony, no doubt used for seasonal orientation and to promote sensory stimulation. A household model of care was also in evidence, with all decision-making about care needs, activities and information shared between staff, residents and family members. This was clearly 'a home from home', where staff were trained and encouraged to undertake 'risk-benefit assessments' and to consider not only the potential danger associated with certain actions proceeding, but also the risks involved should a resident be forbidden from pursuing those actions (Nuffield Council on Bioethics, 2009; Morgan and Andrews, 2016). The unit also had a policy of whenever possible allowing new residents to have their domestic animals such as cats, budgies and small dogs accompany them. Even following a pet owner's death, the pet remained in the unit. Environments like these that are homely, personalized and encourage choice and autonomy, enhance quality of life (Lawton, 2001; Bradshaw et al, 2012; Moyle et al, 2015).

If internal doors are locked, people may feel displaced and at the extreme, trapped inside (Moyle et al, 2015). This issue was well highlighted in a Scandinavian study (Heggestad et al, 2013, p 887),[2] where a policy of locking internal doors, including the staff room and kitchen doors, existed, and where residents were seriously restricted. In this study an elderly lady living with dementia said: "You know it's like a prison without bars.... I feel like a prisoner. I have no freedom." In the same study, another lady diagnosed with dementia, who enjoyed gardening, also felt imprisoned since she was not allowed go out unsupervised. She commented: "Here we don't have the opportunity to go out. I love to go digging in my garden.... We should have the opportunity to go out more but I don't think they [the carers] have time for that. You know I'm just sitting here, that's a little boring."

Kitwood (1997a) pointed to the range of factors, biological, environmental, social, psychological and emotional, that influence the individual's subjective experience of dementia. The manipulation of any of these factors can promote or undermine personhood and contribute to wellbeing or ill-being. The narratives here provide powerful accounts of what it is like for the individual in a care home when connections to former life experiences and current experiences are severed (Bartlett and O'Connor, 2010), and when they are denied the opportunity to pursue lifetime interests (Moyle et al, 2015). The narratives also provide nuanced insights into everyday life inside care homes, how some people construct and perceive reality and how the individual makes sense of their everyday world (Phoenix, 2008). Through this rich qualitative data, we are reminded of how disabling and damaging a physical environment can be, yet how relatively easy and inexpensive it may be to remove some of the artificial barriers (attitudinal and environmental) that cause 'excess disability'.

The way forward

Many 'behaviours that challenge' occur as a result of the person's attempt to communicate their unmet needs (Kitwood, 1997a). Unmet needs, including untreated pain, untreated delirium, infections, hunger, thirst, loneliness, boredom and frustration, can all contribute to 'behaviours that challenge', as can staff's poor understanding of dementia, inadequate communication and their lack of knowledge of the resident's life story and biography (Brooker and Latham, 2016). In the absence of training and in large institutional settings, where care practices are highly routinized, where staff numbers and skill mix are inadequate, the individual is at heightened risk of having their rights threatened or, as noted by Kitwood (1997a, p 135), having their psychological needs 'blanked out with tranquillizing medication.'

Knowing the resident's life story reflects a common humanity (Welford et al, 2010), and supporting the person to build on their retained abilities (Post, 2000) and experience personal growth (Bartlett and O'Connor, 2010) is critical to their wellbeing. Quality of life is about 'knowing the resident' and allowing that person to hold on to their identity, character and even some personal possessions. It is about the small things of care, 'the humanity with which assistance for everyday living is offered ... the manner and tone in which a person is addressed ... and {encouraged to} access meaningful activity' (Nuffield Council on Bioethics, 2009, p 49). Out of fear of litigation, care environments may be designed that provide clinically safe pathways to loneliness, boredom and at the extreme, death.

So far this chapter has explored the way in which chemical and physical restraints, used to address 'behaviours that challenge', can, in some circumstances, be very harmful and can violate an individual's fundamental human rights. Technology is yet another possible solution often used in care homes to address 'behaviours that challenge', and the section that follows briefly discusses this important topic in the context of human rights.

Assistive and surveillance technologies

Technology is a broad concept, covering a whole range of devices often used in dementia care. Assistive technology (AT) (see Chapter Four for a definition) has the potential to provide one possible solution to the multiple challenges dementia poses. Another potential solution is found in surveillance technology (ST), where for example cameras, sensors or alarms are used to monitor and observe. In the context of long-term care and human rights, however, the use of AT and ST is contentious (Alzheimer Europe, 2010; Niemeijer et al, 2010, 2015).

Two general reviews of the AT literature (Topo, 2009; Niemeijer et al, 2010) and a systematic review (Fleming and Sum, 2014) all call for more robust empirical evidence to demonstrate the effectiveness of these technologies in dementia care. Topo's (2009) review of 46 studies showed that the user voice was largely missing in all research endeavours, and the cost-effectiveness of technologies remained unknown. Fleming and Sum's systematic review (2014) of 41 publications demonstrated very weak evidence to support the assumption that technology improves safety for people diagnosed with dementia.

Much AT, especially for those with a mild to moderate dementia, focuses on attempting to promote autonomy, independence and quality of life (Cash, 2003; Hagen et al, 2004; Cahill et al, 2004; Topo et al, 2004; Cheek et al, 2005; Robinson et al, 2009; Alzheimer Europe, 2010). For a person with a more severe dementia, much AT is designed to monitor and promote their safety. Sadly, the use of AT to support cognitive functioning, enhance social contacts and provide opportunities for recreation is fairly limited (Torhild Holthe, personal communication, 2016).

From a human rights perspective, an important consideration is the extent to which AT may reduce or sever human contact as some people who have a severe dementia and live in care homes may already have limited physical contact with others (Nuffield Council on Bioethics, 2009).

Other considerations include the extent to which AT:

- empowers or dehumanizes the individual (Astell, 2006)
- promotes or undermines the resident's personhood and dignity
- increases or decreases autonomy and privacy
- extends or limits self-determination and safety (Hofmann, 2013)

as each of these issues infringe on human rights. In addition, some practical questions need to be raised, such as:

- Who is responsible for the monitoring of the technology?
- How robust and reliable is it?
- How frequently will it need maintenance, repair and upgrading?
- How well are staff trained to use the devices?
- Was consent/assent from the individual diagnosed with dementia sought and obtained? (Torhild Holthe, personal communication, 2017)

Alzheimer Europe (2010) argues that AT should never be used if devices infringe on civil liberties or result in coercion or social control. The main reason for its use should be to benefit the person living with dementia. Prior to use, a comprehensive assessment of risk, need and benefits should be performed (Alzheimer Europe, 2010). If AT is used to control, coerce or restrict freedom, without the person's informed consent, or as a solution for staff shortages (Zwijsen et al, 2011), or to replace human contact, then such practices are unethical and constitute a breach of human rights.

A particularly controversial technological 'solution' often used in care homes for people diagnosed with dementia is 'electronic tagging' (Hughes and Louw, 2002; O'Neill, 2002; Astell, 2006). This term refers to a situation where markers, generally a wrist or ankle bracelet, are attached to a person usually for the purpose of promoting safety and monitoring behaviour. Since the concept of 'tagging' has traditionally been associated with the control and management of thieves and criminals (Bewley, 1998), the language here is dehumanizing. For this reason, a more preferable term, and one chosen for use in Norway, is 'localization technology' (Öderud et al, 2013).

Proponents in favour of 'localization technology' argue that it can promote dignity, independence, personhood and autonomy by offering the individual freedom to move about in a safe, secure physical environment. Indeed, it is claimed that this type of intervention is preferable to locked wards and sedation (Bail, 2003). Yet opponents argue that 'localization technology' strips people of their freedom, undermines autonomy (Landau et al, 2010), and can be dehumanizing since it is associated with criminal behaviour and reflects a surveillance rather than a person-centred ethos (Robinson et al, 2007).

Finding the right balance between a person's rights to positive risk taking, independence and autonomy and a practitioner's duty and responsibility to promote safety and reduce risk is a critical dilemma in decision-making about using AT (Robinson et al, 2007), as is the issue of obtaining consent or assent and the overall ethics of technology use (Bjørneby et al, 2004; Andrews and Robinson, 2013). Irrespective of the level of a person's disability, cognizance needs to be given to the ramifications AT has in terms of human rights (Welsh et al, 2003; Hughes, 2011). The inappropriate use of any form of AT can result in degrading treatment and can seriously interfere with the individual's right to freedom, choice and independence.

In any discussion about human rights dementia and technology, the use of ST such as surveillance cameras, GPS, censors (to detect body temperature, falls, motion and so on) and alarms must also be considered. Boekhorst and colleagues' study (2013) showed that compared with physical restraints, ST had no significant effect on quality of life for people with dementia resident in long-stay residential care. Their work also showed that a person with more advanced dementia was more likely to be physically restrained compared with those who had a milder dementia, where ST tended to be used.

Niemeijer et al's (2010) review, where they investigated the practical and moral appropriateness of using ST in residential care, noted a conflict of interest between those of the institution and residents, and concluded that '... there is a clear lack of consensus on how surveillance technologies can contribute to the quality of care for people with dementia or intellectual disability in an ethically viable way and [our overview] has further pointed to omissions and lack of depth within the ethical debate' (2010, p 1139). These same researchers also highlighted a shortage of resident users' perspectives on the use and usefulness of such technology.

A conclusion reached based on the empirical research reviewed for this chapter is that people with dementia have largely been regarded as passive participants in studies on AT and ST, and that technologies may be more beneficial for family members or nursing home staff than for the individual diagnosed with dementia (Niemeijer et al, 2010; Gibson et al, 2015). Yet despite this finding a strong policy commitment to AT use is enshrined in many countries' national dementia strategies (see DH, 2009; ASPE, 2013; Scottish Government, 2013; Australian Government Department of Health, 2015), and endorsed in the Organisation for Economic Co-operation and Development (OECD) report on dementia (2015). There is a need for much more robust research to be conducted in this area that is inclusive of the voice of the individual using the technology.

Questions that need to be asked include, why is public debate on AT and dementia not more advanced, especially in the context of long-term care? Why is technology so widely promoted in the absence of a solid evidence base (Gibson et al, 2015)? Whose interests are being served by the promotion of AT and ST, in the absence of empirical evidence demonstrating usefulness? This brief critical review reveals that whilst overall technologies can potentially benefit the individual, such solutions may also affront personhood, threaten human rights and contribute to 'excess disability'.

Kitwood argued that any intervention in dementia care should be primarily concerned with the preservation of personhood and with addressing unmet needs (Kitwood, 1997a). Therefore, in using any technology, a starting point should be an analysis of why the device is needed (Marshall, 2003), how can it promote dignity and autonomy and uphold human rights, and what attempt has been made by staff, even when residents have severe dementia, to communicate to them the rationale behind the use of the device (Nuffield Council on Bioethics, 2009).

Support for personal care

Supporting a cognitively impaired person with their personal care needs, including assisting a person to dress, shower, bath, eat and toilet, is an extremely intimate and private matter (Baker, 2015), and the provision of this type of personal support must be done in a way that is not degrading or inhuman, and is respectful of the person's dignity (Nuffield Council on Bioethics, 2009). Knowing the right amount of support to offer requires skill, knowledge, sensitivity, judgement, time and occasionally, positive risk-taking. It may be easier for busy staff to take over completely, doing everything for the individual rather than enabling that person to slowly undertake parts of their own routines by themselves (Brooker and Latham, 2016). By denying the individual opportunities to undertake even minor aspects of their own personal care, such as buttoning cardigans/shirts or tying shoe laces, or by adopting the role of decision-making in every aspect of the individual's life (Parker and Penhale, 1998; O'Connor and Purves, 2009), staff may inadvertently deskill and disempower the resident (Woods, 1999).

Freedom to choose and exercise control over decision-making are important aspects of quality of life for the individual living with a dementia in a care home (Dröes et al, 2006; Crespo et al, 2011; Moyle et al, 2011; O'Rourke et al, 2015). Yet, autonomy (see Chapter Three for a definition) in the context of dementia still tends to be regarded by many as an all-or-nothing concept, and some individuals, because of dementia, are at risk of having all their autonomy rights restricted or removed (Boyle, 2008; O'Connor and Purves, 2009). In this context, the concept of relational autonomy as espoused by the Nuffield Council on Bioethics (2009) (see Chapter Three) is very helpful. This is where autonomy is no longer understood as the ability to make and communicate rational decisions but rather, it is seen in a broader sense to reflect the individual's sense of self and that person's capacity to value one thing over another and express their preferences (Nuffield Council on Bioethics, 2009). Adopting this more nuanced approach to understanding autonomy has much potential to promote a person's quality of life in long-term care.

In terms of personal care, supporting a person to toilet independently may be challenging for care staff, particularly if the individual resists assistance and reacts aggressively, believing that their privacy and personal space is being intruded (Woods, 2001). It is not unusual for some older people to be designated as *incontinent* and given incontinence pads simply because they can no longer walk independently or because the system of care cannot adapt to their complex needs (Alzheimer Europe, 2012). A colleague whose mother had dementia and who recently died in a nursing home discussed with me the fact that her mother was compelled to wear incontinence pads, even though her main health problem was immobility and not incontinence. Commenting on a particular incident that occurred when she requested urgent assistance for her mother but was ignored, she said:

> I think the crux of it is that Mum was treated as *incontinent* even though she was *continent*, but due to the illness she was no longer mobile (and could not get to the bathroom alone). On this particular occasion, when I was visiting with my son, she articulated a need to go to the bathroom and needed assistance. Once Mum became immobile staff told us that *we were not allowed to assist with toileting.* So I sent my son out for the health care assistant who said she would be down in 15 minutes. My Mum kept saying "I don't want to soil the sofa, I don't want to soil the sofa." Anyway she did [soil herself] and it gets even worse as even after she soiled herself, I wheeled Mum down to the care assistant and asked her to take Mum to the bathroom, she said "I told

your son I'll do it in in 15 minutes." Now she [Mum] had piles and fissures; aside from the indignity and inhumanity, she should not have been left sitting like this for medical reasons. (Colleague and daughter of a lady diagnosed with dementia and resident in a nursing home; emphasis added)

Similar acts of omission resulting in degrading, inhuman treatment and physical and psychological humiliation were well articulated in a Scandinavian study (Nåden et al, 2013) when a resident's spouse said:

Needing to go to the toilet at night, one rings the bell and no one comes. Or the health personnel shout that you have to poop in the nappy. I have been shocked several times by the fact that people behave so badly, that nights are like nightmares. I get to know very much from older people who are living at nursing home residences, even from family members who experience that they are not welcome there because they stick their noses into matters. They are looked upon as bothersome in one way or another.... I have been so frustrated over the fact that residents tell that there is no point in calling for help at night; health personnel do not come.... (Wife carer of a nursing home resident, quoted in Nåden et al, 2013, p 754)

Accounts like these reflect inhuman and unethical practices where the individual is treated as a non-person, where regimes are task-centred, not person-centred, and where paid staff lack the human traits that we know are the essence of good quality care (Kennerley and de Waal, 2013) and instead, rush about operating essentially to a check list (McLean, 2007). Sadly such suboptimal practices, which violate human rights, are more likely to occur in care environments where the old culture of care still prevails (Kitwood, 1997a).

An organizational culture that focuses only on delivering the physical tasks of care (Doyle and Rubinstein, 2014) and one that pathologizes people (Boyle, 2008; Sabat, 2014), ignoring their humanity, breaches human rights by assaulting personhood, dignity, integrity and selfhood. Care practices that negate personhood and are disrespectful of dignity (Baldwin and Capstick, 2007) often occur behind closed doors and may not be visible to regulators and inspectors of care homes. They are more likely to occur in organizations that are poorly resourced and those that subscribe to the 'old culture of care'. As noted by Kitwood

(1997a, p 140), 'care is relatively cheap when there is a thorough disregard for personhood.'

The way forward

Policy-makers need to understand that supporting a person with advanced dementia, who is likely to have additional co-morbidities, requires a highly skilled workforce, one proficient in dementia care, in gerontological nursing and in palliative care. Dementia care can be hard physical labour, but it can also be very rewarding (Lawton et al, 1989; Cahill, 1997). It cannot be undertaken cheaply by untrained staff (Brooker and Latham, 2016). There is a need for adequate pay awards, enhanced working conditions and improved career opportunities for all engaged in dementia care (OECD, 2015). There is a need for better recognition of long-term care as a profession with ongoing opportunities for training (OECD, 2015). There is a need for careful recognition of the specific challenges (language and communication) that face migrant care workers given that long-term dementia care services are increasingly being delivered by migrant health professionals and migrant care workers (WHO, 2012).

All health service professionals and care staff need supportive, sensitive mentoring, effective leadership and competency-based training (Brodaty and Cumming, 2010) along with training in human rights (Kelly and Innes, 2012). They also need to be afforded opportunities to implement new learning obtained through training. Training can lead to a reduction in the use of antipsychotic medication (Fossey et al, 2006), a reduction in the use of physical restraints (Muñiz et al, 2016), and can decrease 'behaviours that challenge' (Brooker et al, 2016). Training can also reduce worker stress and improve work performance (Edvardsson et al, 2009), and it can have a positive influence on how staff interact with residents with dementia (Spector et al, 2013). Educational providers need to ensure that dementia is part of all medical nursing and allied health curricula (Kennerly and de Waal, 2013).

So far the chapter has explored the individual's rights to be protected from torture or cruel, inhuman or degrading treatment or punishment. It has demonstrated the vulnerability of some cognitively impaired individuals who, because of 'behaviours that challenge', are at heightened risk of being subjected to discriminatory policies, especially in care environments, which reflect a malignant social psychology (Kitwood, 1997a). The next section of this chapter progresses to exploring Articles 22 (right to privacy) and 9 (right to accessibility).

The right to privacy

A core theme underpinning the earlier discussion in this chapter has been that of autonomy (Boyle, 2008) or the individual's right to self-determination, to choice and control (Murphy and Welford, 2012). But closely related to the concept of autonomy is that of privacy, which, broadly speaking, refers to the ability of people to seclude themselves or information about themselves from others. Privacy is said to be associated with rights to absolute dignity and to be treated respectfully as a human being (Nordenfelt, 2004; Heggestad et al, 2013). For a person living with dementia in a care home, important physical dimensions of privacy include having one's own private bedroom and bathroom, one's personal possessions including clothing, and having one's own 'front door', so to speak, on which outsiders must knock to gain entrance. Privacy rights also include the right not be disturbed or observed by others (McShane et al, 1994).

The Alzheimer Europe (2012) report notes that many residents with dementia eat, wash, socialise, dress, undress and sleep in the same room as other people, and comment that this reflects '... a total lack of privacy and failure to respect individuality and choice' (2012, p 90). This reminds us of how the physical environment plays a key role in promoting or impeding the privacy rights of a person living with dementia (Lawton, 1977, 2001; Pierce et al, 2015), and quality of life in care homes can be enhanced by physical environments that offer individuals their own private bedrooms (Russell et al, 2008; Moyle et al, 2014), facilitate ownership of personal space (Moyle et al, 2015), allow access to private areas outside of bedrooms (Milte et al, 2015) and enable personalization (Mjørud et al, 2017).

The significance of the physical environment in terms of it being used as a therapeutic tool to promote privacy and wellbeing (Lawton, 2001: Marshall, 2001; Pierce et al, 2015) cannot be overestimated. It is next to impossible for a person diagnosed with dementia, living in a care home, to have their rights to privacy respected in a large, busy, noisy Nightingale ward, where sleeping quarters are shared, where noise is rife and where no quiet room is available to facilitate private conversation or to accommodate a person's desire for solitude. Likewise in the absence of an en suite bedroom, it is next to impossible for staff to maintain a resident's privacy, modesty and dignity, particularly if the individual is incontinent or needs extensive support with toileting. Good environmental design is as vital to resident care as nursing care or the approach to the organization of care used within the setting (Calkins, 1988). Respecting a person's privacy rights is much easier in small-scale, home-like environments (Marshall, 1998) that offer individual en suite bedrooms, separate rooms for separate functions, and where small groups of people live together in a household model of care (Verbeek, 2011).

Whilst across the world recent decades have witnessed significant changes to models of long-term care for individuals living with dementia (Verbeek et al, 2009; Verbeek, 2011, 2013; Black and Rabins, 2013), with the emphasis today being placed on small-scale, home-like residential care models (Ausserhofer et al, 2016), where values of autonomy, the preservation of the individual's self identity, personhood, privacy and collective decision-making are promoted (Verbeek, 2013), the reality is that globally, only a small proportion of people will ever gain access to such models of long-term care (de Lange et al, 2011; Harris-Kojetin et al, 2013). Indeed, most long-term care for people living with dementia is not purpose-built or designed to cater for their usually complex needs. Because of this, most people will have no choice except to live in generic residential care homes, where staff are likely to have heavy workloads and where quality of care may be compromised (Murphy et al, 2006) and privacy rights may be completely overlooked.

Whilst innovative models of long-term care that promote quality of life (including respect for privacy) have been endorsed by organizations including the WHO, International Association of Gerontology and Geriatrics and Institute of Medicine in the US (Ausserhofer et al, 2016), and whilst most of the national dementia strategies reviewed for this book contain compelling messages about the importance of quality of life in long-stay residential care, with some few exceptions (see Australian Government Department of Health, 2015; Norwegian Government, 2016) most fail to explicitly promote household models of long-stay care and none, to my knowledge, set down any targets regarding the provision of SCUs. This is despite the fact that research, although still at an early stage, has shown many benefits associated with such models (Zeisel et al, 2003; Reimer et al, 2004; Cadigan et al, 2012; Bobersky, 2013; Verbeek, 2013; Ausserhofer et al, 2016).

Household models of long-term care are in keeping with the reablement approach to the support of people living with dementia introduced in Chapter Four. They are also well aligned with WHO's conceptualization of disability as reflected in the ICF and discussed in Chapter Two. The reablement approach leads to a consideration of the contextual factors (personal and environmental) likely to impact on the subjective experience and on individual strengths, retained abilities and what people can do that is important to them. It reflects a shift from biomedical frameworks that are task-driven and that ignore subjectivity, to person-centred holistic frameworks that are value-driven and focus on wellbeing and empowerment (WHO, 2012), and where the individual is supported to live well in a purpose-built environment, assisted by well-trained staff.

Advocacy groups including the DAI, Alzheimer Societies, the ADI and civil society need to place more pressure on governments to provide realistic funding for the expansion of more innovative household models of long-term care. More research is needed that builds on theoretical grounds and that incorporates comparative research methods examining multiple outcomes for both the resident, family member and staff (Ausserhofer et al, 2016). In particular, robust studies that provide evidence of the cost-effectiveness of more innovative models of long-term care are needed as to date, this type of data is lacking (Hilda Verbeek, personal communication, 2017).

The right to access the physical environment

Imagine you are a farmer and have spent your life strolling around country fields, chasing stray animals, and in your leisure time, fishing on the nearby lakes. Now you are 80 years old and have recently been admitted to a care home where you are surrounded by other residents, most of whom are women. They spend their time indoors playing bingo, perhaps going to mass, to exercise classes, getting their hair done and participating in the weekly quiz. You are not religious, you were never particularly sociable and you hate all of these activities. Your bedroom overlooks a large field with cattle grazing down by a lake – you yearn to go out, access fresh air, and although you repeatedly ask, you are told you must remain indoors since staff are 'too busy' to accompany you outside. How might you feel, and if you became frustrated, how might this be interpreted? The scenario here may not be that unusual. Indeed, boredom and frustration may be the reality for some elderly men living with dementia in long-term care facilities today, where the care environment tends to be female-dominated, and where activity programmes are not always gender-sensitive.

A care home is a building that extends into its nearby local community (Milte et al, 2016), and it should never be assumed that once admitted the individual becomes socially disconnected from the rest of the world (Nuffield Council on Bioethics, 2009). Indeed, wherever possible, a person should be given opportunities for social engagement and supported to access local amenities including cafes, shops, churches, parks, town halls, cinemas and so on. Access to the physical environment is important, not least for physical exercise, contact with nature, sensory stimulation and the execution of the normal activities of daily living (Girardet and Schumacher, 1999; Pollock, 2001; Timlin and Rysenbry, 2010; Pollock and Marshall, 2012). A policy whereby residents have the freedom to go outside and access outdoor space should be written into the care philosophy of every long-term care environment (Welsh et al, 2003).

Importantly, every care home should have a safe, secure, multisensory garden that is easily accessible to residents, even those with mobility problems. Fresh air is important for the regulation of circadian rhythms and sleep–wake patterns (Brawley, 2001), for the enjoyment of nature and seasonal orientation (Gilliard and Marshall, 2012), and for a change of ambience (Cohen and Weisman, 1991). Much research evidence now exists showing the multiple benefits of well-designed gardens (Pollock and Marshall, 2012), including exposure to natural light (Calkins et al, 2007), reminiscence (Jarrott et al, 2002), physical activities (Lindenmuth and Moose, 1990) and contact with outdoor greenery, and how access to the physical environment can support competence in people living with dementia (Rappe and Topo, 2007). The ongoing absence of access to outdoor areas for people resident in long stay residential care breaches human rights. Even prisoners are allowed regular access to outdoor areas (Alzheimer Europe, 2012).

Right to participate in meaningful activities

In this final part of the chapter, the extent to which the individual's right to participate in cultural, recreational and leisure-time activities, in residential care facilities is explored. How people spend their time in care homes impacts on their quality of life and cultural recreational and leisure-time activities, (Article 30) collectively referred to for the purpose of this chapter as *meaningful activities*, are well-known and important aspects of quality of life (Train et al, 2005; Harmer and Orrell, 2008; Cahill and Diaz-Ponce, 2011; Diaz-Ponce and Cahill, 2013; Theurer et al, 2015; Milte et al, 2016; Mjørud et al, 2017).

A broad range of activities can be used to promote the quality of life of people living with dementia in care homes. Examples include reminiscence therapy, which involves discussions of former activities and experiences, either individually or in group sessions (Gibson, 2011; Parsons, 2015); music therapy, where trained therapists use music actively or passively to trigger memories and sensations (Fang et al, 2017); cognitive stimulation therapy, a group-based activity targeting social and cognitive functioning (Clare and Woods, 2004); aromatherapy, where pure fragrant plant oils are used to help relieve health problems (Forrester et al, 2014); doll therapy, a sometimes controversial intervention used to reduce anxiety and improve communication (Mitchell and Templeton, 2014); and Snoezelens (Chung and Lai, 2002), or multisensory stimulation, where triggers such as music, bubble tubes and projected imagery are used for psychosocial stimulation (Brooker, 2001).

Some of these interventions have been the subject of systematic reviews and careful evaluation, and emerging evidence demonstrates largely positive results (see for example Spector et al, 2000, 2006, 2011; Burns et al, 2005; Woods et al, 2005; Coen et al, 2011, Beard, 2012). Other activities used in long-stay care facilities include pet therapy, creative therapies such as art and pottery work, dance, computer games and structured activity programmes including physical exercise. In terms of activities, what is critically important is not so much their range, but rather, their quality (Theurer et al, 2015), and the extent to which they are 'meaningful' to the individual and contribute to that person's quality of life.

All of the national dementia strategies critically reviewed for this book reflect a strong commitment to improving quality of life for the individual living with dementia in long-term care (see, for example, Objective 5 of the French national plan for 'Alzheimer and related diseases' (2008-2012), Ministry of Health (France), 2008;[3] and Objective 11 of England's Living well with dementia: A national dementia strategy, DH, 2009 and Section 10 of Northern Ireland's regional strategy, DHSSPS, 2011). The WHO (2012) report also reflects a firm commitment to improving long-term residential care, and for guidelines on long-term care to be developed that 'should include guidance on the provision of social engagement and recreational activities, cognitive stimulation and rehabilitation ... and environments that are both safe and stimulating...' (WHO, 2012, p 63). Yet despite the rhetoric of government policy, evidence emerging even in countries boasting national dementia strategies is that there is scope to significantly improve quality of life and to transform recreational opportunities for residents who have dementia.

For example, a UK Alzheimer's Society report (2013b[4]) noted that less than half (41 per cent) of 'family caregivers' believed that their relative's quality of life in care homes was good, and only 44 per cent of family members rated opportunities for activities as good. In a Northern Ireland study that explored the human rights of older people in nursing homes (Northern Ireland Human Rights Commission,

2012), findings revealed how nursing home staff were not committed to ensuring the human rights of older people were upheld. The study also found that insufficient emphasis was placed on 'set activities and events and opportunities to go outdoors ... and [enable the residents to] have regular interaction with staff' (Northern Ireland Human Rights Commission, 2012, p 33). The need for staff training, more adequate staffing, better record keeping, especially in the context of drug use and antipsychotic medication, and attention to personal care activities were some of the deficits highlighted in this report.[5]

A small but rich evidence base is also slowly emerging, reflecting first-person accounts of quality of life in care homes including residents' views on activity programmes (see, for example, Moyle et al, 2011; Cahill and Diaz-Ponce, 2011; O'Rourke et al, 2015). By and large, findings support those reported in commissioned reports. In Norway, for example, Mjørud and colleagues (2017) have recently shown that across three nursing homes investigated, residents diagnosed with dementia reported that most activities were boring and they found their days monotonous. Some slept through activities, and the continuation of former hobbies known to be important for preserving personhood (Palmer, 2013) and that may have enhanced their quality of life were sometimes overlooked.

Meaningful activities need not necessarily be 'therapeutic' and 'domestic activities' such as helping others by doing odd jobs can also give pleasure and promote quality of life (Moyle et al, 2015). In a study referenced earlier by Nåden and colleagues (2013), some poignant examples were given of the type of activities some residents clearly enjoyed but that they were forbidden from pursuing, including, in one case, a person not being allowed to listen to music because staff believed that this could cause distress. One of the most powerful examples cited in this same study of how a 'domestic activity' (helping fellow residents in the dining room) was stopped and how stopping this 'meaningful activity' led to the resident's 'excess disability' was provided by a daughter, who said:

> My father liked the small dining room at the ward, but he had to leave it quite quickly. He summoned the personnel too much. He cared much for the other residents and called for the personnel when they dropped things, [on floor] and then he was not allowed to sit there anymore and was moved to the kitchen where those who are most sick are placed. He became so anxious about that, looking at them sitting in their wheelchairs. He became worse after that. There

should be an alternative – one of the personnel could be nearby and help them while they are eating. (daughter of man with dementia, Nåden et al, 2013, p 754)

More attention needs to be focused in care homes on choice in relation to activity participation and on the potential contribution social relationships can make to residents' wellbeing. In this context, Theurer and colleagues' (2015) work, where they call for a cultural revolution to occur in nursing homes, is very relevant. They claim that there is a rich reservoir of untapped talent and stimuli available amongst residents with dementia in long-term care settings, and suggest that 'recreational activities' needs to be replaced with 'resident engagement and peer support programmes' designed by and for the resident. In their view, even residents with an advanced dementia can benefit from such engagement. Programmes like these, designed to return power and control back to the resident and promote autonomy, are laudable and may be more engaging and pleasurable than fitting the person into pre-existing, rigidly scheduled activities considered by some as boring. However, what is not discussed in their work are the resources needed, including the training required to motivate and upskill frontline care staff to engage in positive risk-taking, promote resident autonomy and facilitate these types of creative programmes which, if they go wrong, could have adverse consequences.

The right to meaningful activities for those with severe dementia

Those residents most likely to have their human rights seriously affronted in care homes are men and women with severe dementia, the majority of whom are extremely frail, functionally dependent, bed-bound (Cadigan et al, 2012) and may no longer be able to talk (Post, 2000). Our own research showed that among men and women who had severe dementia there was a distinct absence of awareness of the activity programmes available within the homes, and most of these people were either indifferent or not interested in discussing the topic of activities (Cahill and Diaz-Ponce, 2011). Instead, what was meaningful for them, as their '… horizons of experience narrow[ed]' (Post, 2000, p 135), were small pleasures such as 'cups of tea, cigarette smoking, a sunny day, the odd chat, or someone giving me an ice cream…' (Cahill and Diaz-Ponce, 2011, p 567). Loneliness, including a desire to 'go home', and at the extreme, a feeling of being abandoned and a quest for human contact, was a striking sub-theme found in the rich qualitative data collected from these twenty eight residents with severe dementia.

Although in many cases the voice of the individual is likely to be muted or disjointed at the most disabling stages of dementia (Post, 2000), it needs to be remembered that the person remains an emotional and relational human being (Hughes, 2011), who can still track conversation with an emotional component (Theurer, 2012), and can still exercise agency through non-verbal communication, such as '... vocalizations, grimaces, emotional tone and so forth' (Hughes, 2014, p 190). In other words, personhood still remains right into severe dementia (Hughes, 2014), and even when all language skills are deficient, every effort should be made by staff and family members to understand, encourage and enhance communication (Nuffield Council on Bioethics, 2009) and promote that person's dignity (UNECE, 2015b).

Yet there is a tendency for some relatives and staff to assume that because the person with end-stage dementia can no longer communicate verbally, the only support needed is good medical nursing and clinical care (Hughes, 2014). The perils of treating a person with severe dementia as 'socially dead' (Sweeting and Gilhooley, 1997), simply because their language skills are severely impaired, was well illustrated in Diaz-Ponce's study (2008) of quality of life and dementia. Commenting about how critically important it is for care staff to promote personhood, enhance dignity and provide more than just physical clinical care to a person with a very severe dementia, a daughter said:

> What I think is important for her at the moment is human contact, physical contact, and being talked to. Even if you [the resident] can't talk, you talk back to the person. So it's physical contact, its warmth, and all of that kind of stuff....
> I mean she has to be – medically, she has to be well looked after. But actually no, the top of my list would be contact with people and just nonsense chat and all that kind of stuff. (Daughter of person with severe dementia in long term care, quoted in Diaz-Ponce, 2008, p 65)

In the same study, another family member whose relative had very severe dementia gave a similar account. In this case the emphasis was on multisensory stimulation and the need for specialist activities to be available that might promote personhood. She said:

> ... I think they do some sort of massage and that's alright, but maybe I'd like ... some sort of like reflexology or something that would make contact with the person.... To draw them out. I mean any physical contact is very important, really, when I think in that stage, when you can't talk to anybody. You've got to make that person ... anything; it's the only thing that you've got to work with her. You know they should organize more things for people at this stage. Anything, like the reflexology, anything. (Daughter of person with severe dementia in long term care, quoted in Diaz-Ponce, 2008, p 103)

Post (2000, p 61) notes that in the biomedical model, the emphasis on *'doing to* is sometimes easier than the more appropriate *being with'* and narratives such as these remind us of the phenomenon of *social death*, where the body is biologically alive but the person is treated as socially dead (Sweeting and Gilhooley, (1997) simply because some of their valued attributes, in this case, language skills, are very severely impaired. The data remind us that the loss of verbal skills should never justify the severance of human relationships. Relating to a person as if they no longer exist, as purely a body to be managed, treating the person with social disregard (Brannelly, 2011) and offering that person no sensory stimulation affronts dignity, is discriminatory, and constitutes a serious breach of human rights.

The work of Cohen-Mansfield and colleagues (2011) has demonstrated that remaining occupied has a positive impact on the wellbeing of those whose dementia is advanced, and a variety of different stimuli (live and simulated) can increase levels of engagement. People with severe/advanced dementia can respond to a 'soothing environment: they have aesthetic sense' (Hughes, 2014, p 149). Although maintaining communication with people with severe dementia can be challenging (Allan and Killick, 2008), momentary pleasures, such as a slow hand massage, finger food and actions rather than activities, may be needed (Perrin and May, 2000). Although methodologically challenging there is a need for a lot more research to be conducted with people who have advanced dementia.

Conclusion

This chapter has explored a selection of human rights that are relevant to many individuals diagnosed with dementia who live in care homes. By exploring these topics in the context of the research evidence, I have argued that government policies are, for the most part, failing this very vulnerable group of people whose human rights are often not respected. A key problem highlighted is that many care homes are not purpose-built or customized to accommodate the complex needs of the individual diagnosed with dementia, and non-nursing staff may receive limited dementia-specific training. They may have to work long shifts, they may be poorly paid and may sometimes receive limited support. The provision of quality, individualized, person-centred care for residents with dementia necessitates significant set-up costs and intensive, continuous resourcing and revenue. Advocacy groups must exert pressure on governments to apportion more realistic funding to support quality dementia-specific residential care.

This chapter has also shown that the biomedical model for understanding and responding to dementia prevails, and many people continue to live in long term care settings that are dominated by an excessive focus on clinical management, on drug treatments and on policies of control and restriction. Advocacy groups also need to challenge health reimbursement policies that may help to sustain the biomedical model. Introducing a new conceptual lens and viewing dementia care practice and policy through the compass of human rights helps to highlight some of the injustices, discrimination and harmful practices many individuals diagnosed with dementia are at heightened risk of being exposed to. This same human rights lens and the tools provided in the CRPD can provide the necessary instruments required to campaign for both policy and practice reform. These important issues are discussed in more detail in the chapter that follows.

Summary of key points

- People diagnosed with moderate to severe dementia living in care homes can be exceptionally vulnerable.
- The excessive and unethical use of chemical restraints in care homes constitutes a serious breach of the individual's human rights.
- The unethical and inappropriate use of physical restraints also constitutes a serious breach of human rights.
- Although AT and ST hold promise in terms of promoting the individual's safety and autonomy and contributing to an improved quality of life, depending on how they are used, these technologies may also violate human rights.
- Irrespective of the scale of violation, any human rights breach can be serious as it can result in lasting psychological harm.
- Dementia care is hard, physical and emotional work that cannot be undertaken cheaply by untrained staff.

- Most long-term care facilities are not purpose-built nor designed to address the complex and unique needs of people diagnosed with dementia.
- Autonomy, choice, control and participation in decision-making are critical components of quality of life for people living in care homes.
- Many environmental and attitudinal barriers leading to 'excess disability' could be readily removed at no great expense.
- At the most disabling stages of dementia, where language skills are no longer apparent, the person continues to exist and can still respond to sensory stimuli.
- Educational providers must ensure that dementia is part of all medical, nursing and allied health curricula, and students should gain real-life exposure to people diagnosed with dementia.
- More research that is inclusive of the voice of the individual is needed to gain a better understanding of the important issues that are relevant to the lives of people living with dementia in care homes.

Notes

[1] The term 'care home' is used throughout this chapter to refer to nursing homes and care homes.

[2] It is important to point out that this study provided examples of both good and poor practice, and this particular paper refers only to the latter.

[3] This was the original first French dementia plan. Since that time three further iterations of a French plan have been published.

[4] Findings from an earlier report (Alzheimer's Society, 2007) showed an absence of social interaction and meaningful activities and a lack of dignity and respect for residents with dementia. Half of the family caregivers interviewed for this same study reported that their relatives had insufficient stimulation in care homes. Over a six-hour period, it was noted that a typical resident only spent two minutes interacting with other residents or staff (Alzheimer's Society, 2007).

[5] It is worth noting that care standards for nursing homes in Northern Ireland are now underpinned by both the Human Rights Act and the *European Convention on Human Rights*. In these standards specific reference is made to rights to protection from torture, to privacy and to life.

SIX

Emerging public policy on dementia: the implications of a human rights-based approach for policy and practice

Introduction

The purpose of this chapter is threefold. First it aims to outline those global and European events that have led to the development of public policy on dementia during the last decade. Here it is argued that as a policy area, dementia has only recently been prioritized (Milne, 2010; Wortmann, 2013). And whilst in the past dementia policy lacked clinical and political ownership (Banerjee, 2013), and straddled several different governmental departments (Manthorpe and Adams, 2003), often cross-cutting the boundaries of ageing and mental health policy (Marshall, 1999), nowadays, many countries are developing their own dementia-specific policies (WHO, 2012, 2016; Pot and Petrea, 2013; OECD, 2015) designed to address the significant challenge dementia poses. This part of the chapter briefly reviews a selection of national dementia strategies that are available in English. It shows how a rights-based discourse is gradually beginning to penetrate some, but not all, of these newly developed strategies.

The second part of the chapter advances to a discussion from a human rights-based perspective of practice-based issues in dementia care. It commences by presenting recent data on dementia and human rights collected from a survey of health service professionals and care staff. Based on these findings, it argues for the need for practitioners to be upskilled in human rights principles and legislation.

The third and final part of the chapter raises some critical questions for practitioners relating to equality and justice concerns, and attempts to interrogate dementia care practice by applying human rights principles to everyday, real-life situations. In this final section some synergies are drawn between elements of person-centred care practice (Brooker and Latham, 2016) and human rights principles.

Public policy on dementia

Policy-makers have a growing interest in dementia (Quaglio et al, 2016; Wu et al, 2016), which is now regarded as a key challenge of the 21st century (Wortmann, 2013). Rising prevalence rates combined with the burgeoning cost of dementia and delays in finding a cure (Winblad et al, 2016) are likely to have fuelled this interest. In the past, public policy on dementia fell between the cracks of policies for older people and mental health policy (O'Shea and O'Reilly, 1999), and was often tacked on to both these areas (Manthorpe and Adams, 2003). In the absence of rational planning (Cantley and Smith, 2001), individuals living with dementia were not 'treated as a special and separate group for policy purposes' (Cantley, 2001, p 219). More commonly known as 'senility', and those experiencing the symptoms as 'doting' or 'elderly mentally infirm', the early development of dementia policy, underpinned by the biomedical model, reflected paternalistic approaches including disempowerment and at the extreme, custodial care (McLean, 2010).

Nowadays, improvements in our understanding of dementia, including its current and future financial impact (Wimo et al, 2013; ADI, 2015 estimates suggest that the cost of dementia will reach US$1 trillion worldwide by 2018), have led governments to address its diverse challenges by developing specific policies. Likewise data on current and future incidence and prevalence rates (ADI, 2015a; Wu et al, 2015; Winblad et al, 2016) has probably further precipitated this interest. Although in terms of policy development Australia has trailblazed the world, its first national dementia plan being published in 1992 (Hunter and Doyle, 2014), within Europe, France, led by Nicolas Sarkozy in 2006, laid the foundation for a European dementia policy (Georges, 2013).

European dementia policy

A useful starting point in tracking dementia policy development across Europe is Alzheimer Europe's *Paris Declaration on Dementia* (2006). This document highlighted 19 key priority areas, straddling social, legal, ethical and medical concerns. The *Paris Declaration* called for dementia to be made:

• a public health priority
• for increased research funding to be allocated to dementia
• for compulsory dementia training for medical students

- for EU research collaboration on dementia and
- for governments to develop national dementia strategies (Georges, 2013).

It was strategic politically since it provided the impetus and guidelines for Alzheimer Europe to raise awareness of dementia amongst members of the European Parliament (Georges, 2013). It also acted as a springboard for dementia to be made a key priority area during France's 2008 presidency of the EU. Unsurprisingly, then, a few years after the *Paris Declaration* was launched, in 2009, and as noted by Georges (2013) the European Parliament responded to Sarkozy's plan by launching its *Written Declaration* on dementia (EPWD, 2009)

This *Written Declaration*, which attracted the signatories of 456 members of the European Parliament, called on the Commission, the Council and the governments of member states to acknowledge Alzheimer's disease as a public health priority, and to develop a European action plan on dementia. It formed the genesis for both the Joint Programme for Neurodegenerative Diseases (JPND, 2017) and the European Initiative on Alzheimer's disease (European Parliament, 2011), an initiative that during its initial phase identified four core areas for community action, one of which was 'rights, autonomy and dignity'.

Since 2009, a series of other key legacy events[1] and declarations have occurred, some with a focus on human rights that have helped place dementia on the global and European political agenda. The most notable of these include:

- The UN General Assembly's (2011) *Political declaration of the High-level Meeting of the General Assembly on the prevention and control of non-communicable diseases*, where dementia was identified as an important cause of morbidity, and where equitable access to healthcare interventions was recognized.
- WHO's (2012) report on dementia, *Dementia: A public health priority*, which argued that dementia should be part of the *public health* agenda for all countries, and that worldwide, dementia should be a national public health and social care priority.
- The G8 summit (2013), where a commitment was made to doubling the amount of research funding allocated to dementia and finding a cure by 2025.
- The World Dementia Council (2014), established to draw together international expertise, stimulate innovation and coordinate

international efforts to attract new sources of finance to fund vital dementia research.

- Alzheimer Europe's *Glasgow Declaration* (2014b), where an NGO commitment to promoting the *rights, dignity and autonomy* of people living with dementia was given. It was signed by 11,613 people, 153 policy-makers and 84 MEPs. A commitment was made to develop a European dementia strategy.

- WHO's (2015b) *First ministerial conference on global action against dementia*. The conference was strongly underpinned by *human rights principles*. Eleven key actions were identified that were endorsed by representatives from 89 countries around the world.

- Dementia Forum X (2015), supported by her Majesty Queen Silvia of Sweden, is a global initiative established to take action on dementia and target the unmet needs of those individuals affected by the condition, by engaging business, political, academic and other leaders of society to shape worldwide, regional and industrial agendas. Meetings take place once every two years in Stockholm, and are attended by her Majesty Queen Silvia.

Undoubtedly such declarations and legacy events have played an important role in encouraging countries to develop their own policy plans, and at the time of writing (2017), a total of 26 national dementia strategies[2] have been developed (Batsch, 2016), with some countries, including Australia, France,[3] Denmark, Scotland and the US, now on to their third and in the case of France fourth strategies/updates.

Ten key policy objectives are common across these national dementia strategies (ADI, 2013; Wortmann, 2013), all of which are underpinned by a commitment to personhood (O'Shea et al, 2015), to living well with dementia (DH, 2009) and to improving quality of care (Fortinsky and Downs, 2014). With a central focus on early diagnosis and interventions, a biomedical focus was evident in the earlier strategies as, for example, in the English *Living well with dementia: A national dementia strategy* (DH, 2009), where a priority was placed on memory clinic expansion, and in the third French strategy, *French national plan for 'Alzheimer and related diseases' (2008-2012)*, Ministry of Health (France), 2008), where the management of the 'behavioural and psychological symptoms of dementia' was a key focus.

More recently, however, this biomedical focus is less dominant, and dementia is being increasingly framed as a public health issue (WHO, 2012), and as both a human rights and public health issue (WHO, 2016). What is missing, particularly from most of the earlier strategies (Australia, Finland, Northern Ireland and Argentina being exceptions), is a focus on risk reduction,[4] and on the important links between healthy lifestyle maintenance and primary prevention. What is also missing is the inclusion of Alzheimer's disease in countries' other national policies such as health promotion policies and policies on preventive health (Travers et al, 2015).

The policy process

How policy on dementia is formulated warrants brief consideration since its development is complex (Banerjee, 2013; Quaglio et al, 2016). It is often assumed that research plays a major role, and that there is a linear relationship between quality research, public awareness and government policy (Prince, 2015). Yet, in the real world, this is rarely the case (Marshall, 1999), particularly when policy-makers are busy, likely to be influenced by different knowledge sources (Hammersley, 2014; Quaglio et al, 2016), and may be under political pressure from different interest groups.

Given how the individual living with dementia and their family members will ultimately be the main beneficiaries of policies, their involvement is critical (Pot and Petrea, 2013), as they are the experts to whom we need to listen (Eley, 2016). Yet evidence suggests that their views have not always been consistently sought. For example, although The Alzheimer Society of Ireland was represented on the government's working group, leading to the development of *The Irish national dementia strategy* (DoH, 2014), it was their CEO and not a person living with dementia or a family member who sat at the table. Likewise in the original English national dementia strategy (DH, 2009), during the consultation phase, only 19 of the 600 responses (3 per cent) came from people living with dementia (McCabe and Bradley, 2012).

It is also important to consider how user engagement is employed and constructed. If the dominant discourse is that of rights and citizenship, norms of social justice are likely to be realized, and user engagement will be framed as a way of ensuring that those most acutely affected by the policy have been active participants in decision-making. Such engagement can result in a real shift in the balance of power relations (Smith et al, 2012). However, if a consumer discourse is dominant, where the user is viewed as the customer, meaningful participation cannot be achieved since the approach fails to address the imbalance of power and divergences of interest between users and providers of services (Lewis, 2009). Supply-side concerns and organizational procedures and practices will likely dominate the relationship.

Ultimately, decision-making about policy priorities is highly political (Gardner and Barraclough, 1992), tokenism may creep into the policy process, and the user voice may be suppressed and far from equal with that of the voice of more powerful interest groups/stakeholders (Lewis, 2009). Eventually decisions about who gets what in terms of resource allocation may be more strongly influenced by those groups that are the most highly organized (Quaglio et al, 2016) and those with the most political and economic power (Cantley and Smith, 2001), including senior ministers, politicians and civil servants, and funding sources including the Exchequer and philanthropic and pharmaceutical companies (Banerjee, 2013), rather than by the agendas of consumer groups. Naturally when the user voice is ignored, policies may not be that relevant to the everyday life of those for whom they are designed (Eley, 2016).

Earlier chapters in this book have shown how current policies targeting the individual living with dementia at home or in care homes are not always relevant to their lives (Clarke et al, 2013; Bökberg et al, 2015). This is probably because the user's voice has not traditionally been sought out or listened to, and because policy-makers tend to hold a deficit view of dementia, conceptualizing it in terms of dependency, costs and residential care (O'Shea et al, 2015), and not in terms of independence, autonomy and quality of life. It may also be because user engagement is often a one-off event (Eley, 2016) rather than a cumulative process, where users remain engaged in the entire policy process, and where there is full and equal partnership (Lewis, 2009). If policy is to be relevant to the lives of individuals diagnosed with dementia and their family members, then policy-makers need to listen to what matters most to them.

Needs are not constant for long in dementia, so services and supports should be flexible, agile, individualized and the views of the user should be sought. The Healthbridge report (Clarke et al, 2013), which captured the user's voice after new, individualized and flexible services were introduced in certain areas in the UK, investigated the usefulness of peer support networks and dementia adviser service supports. The evaluation showed that the individual living with dementia and their family members welcomed new services over traditional ones, since the new interventions empowered many individuals to regain a sense of normality following diagnosis, helped to avert problems and supported individuals in their decision-making (Clarke et al, 2013).

Since the time of their trial, similar approaches to dementia services have been rolled out through the Dementia Engagement & Empowerment Project (DEEP) (Eley, 2016). However, without user engagement and service evaluation, nothing may have happened to shift this direction in service supports. Irish-based research that evaluated new models of respite care yielded similar results (Cahill et al, 2014a), where it was shown that what mattered most to the individual was that interventions were flexible, person-centred and empowering, and that staff were well trained, reliable and respectful.

Service transformation is not possible through one-off interventions or events. It is an iterative process requiring the ongoing engagement of all stakeholders, information networks and meaningful evaluation of process, impact and outcomes. Given the recent trend towards framing dementia as a human rights concern (Kelly and Innes, 2012; Mental Health Foundation, 2015; Bryden, 2015; Rees, 2015; WHO, 2015a; DAI, 2016; Swaffer, 2016), to what extent do national dementia strategies take cognizance of human rights?

Underpinning national dementia strategies with rights-based principles

Based on a perusal of 10 countries' national dementia strategies, a conclusion reached is that whilst some countries' policy plans as, for example, Scotland (*Scotland's national dementia strategy (2013-2016)*, Scottish Government, 2013), Norway (*Dementia plan* 2020, Norwegian Government, 2016), the US (*National plan to address Alzheimer's disease: 2016 update*, ASPE, 2016) and Australia (*National framework for action on dementia 2015-2019*, Australian Government Department of Health, 2015), fare well in terms of reflecting a moderately strong commitment to human rights principles, other countries including Switzerland (*Swiss national dementia strategy 2014-2019*, Federal Office of Public Health (Switzerland), 2016), Ireland (*The Irish national dementia strategy*, DoH, 2014), Malta (*A national strategy for dementia in the Maltese islands, 2015-2023*, Malta, 2015), Gibraltar (*National dementia vision and strategy for Gibraltar*, HM Government of Gibraltar, 2015) and Israel (*National Programme for Addressing Alzheimer's and other types of dementia: Israeli national strategy*, INS, 2013) fare badly.

Noteworthy here is the fact that where reference to human rights occurs in strategy documents, the emphasis is largely on 'civil and political rights' such as the right to respect, dignity, non-discrimination, safety and autonomy, and not on 'social rights' such as the right to welfare services and social care. Likewise, where reference to rights occurs in other international policy documents (see, for example, ADI, *World Alzheimer reports*, 2010-15; ADI, 2015b; WHO, 2012, 2015a; UNECE, 2015a, 2015b), the emphasis again is on negative as opposed to positive rights. The third Scottish strategy (*Scotland's national dementia strategy (2017-2020)*) is an exception here as it provides a useful example of a policy plan firmly committed to respecting and fulfilling positive rights, such as the right to a link worker and to be guaranteed one year of support services following diagnosis. This is not entirely surprising since positive rights such as the right to personal budgets or direct payments (Laybourne et al, 2016) or independent living with personalized supports are resource-intensive (Quinn, 2009), and in the context of the CRPD, not immediately enforceable.

What is being argued here is that although some countries' strategies are now underpinned by rights-based principles, and whilst choice (Boyle, 2010) and consumer-directed care (Tilly and Rees, 2007; Low et al, 2012; Rees, 2015) have become buzz words in some disability and dementia policy debates, the reality is that in most countries, there is a veritable absence of choice available to the individual to exercise their social and economic rights. With reference to the English national dementia strategy (DH, 2009), Boyle (2010, p 517) notes, 'there is a lack of commitment in government policy more generally to providing social care which will enable people with dementia to exercise their human rights to liberty and self-determination.' Her statement could be applied to most countries' national dementia strategies that remain rather vague on social and economic rights. A way forward, although clearly requiring resources, would be to reframe public policy on dementia by using the CRPD and WHO's recent (2016) global action plan on dementia.

Reframing dementia policy with a rights-based approach

Building on O'Shea and colleagues' work (2015, p 110), which proposes a policy frame that replaces the 'individual with collective, biological with social, risk with capabilities, institution with home, deficit with asset and exclusion with inclusion', this new, rights-based policy frame replaces 'marginalization' with 'equality', 'discrimination' with 'participation', 'inequity' with 'social justice' and 'incompetence' with 'personhood'. As noted earlier, in other areas of policy development, particularly in the disability sector (see Chapter Two), service user movements have been instrumental in bringing about change in decision-making and in legislation, policy and service provision (Smith et al, 2012). There is no reason why dementia activists, including the DAI and the Scottish, Irish and European Working Groups, along with the wider dementia community including Alzheimer Europe and the ADI, cannot be successful in transforming the balance of power in dementia interactions and relationships. But this type of change requires honesty, a level playing field, engagement and relationships of trust to be developed between all stakeholders.

So what might a rights-based approach to dementia policy look like? As a start, it would mean all activities related to dementia policy would be underpinned by a strong equalities-based approach (WHO, 2015a; Shakespeare et al, 2017). It would mean more extensive and less tokenistic user engagement with consumer groups. It would mean putting mechanisms in place to ensure that all individuals affected by dementia, irrespective of age, gender, class, education, or ethnicity, would, with the appropriate support from trusted family members be empowered to have their views represented in all policies directly affecting their lives. It would mean that throughout the entire illness trajectory, information about both pharmacological and non-pharmacological interventions would be readily available to the individual and family members.

As shown in Chapter Four, today, an almost carte blanche policy exists to promote early diagnosis and prescribe early drug treatments (cholinesterase inhibitors), but a similar drive to promote non-pharmacological interventions, some of which have been shown to be as cost-effective and clinically effective as drug therapy (ADI, 2011; Knapp et al, 2013), is not in evidence. A rights-based approach would also mean that a broad range of long-term care options, including housing with care models, group living, nursing homes, care homes and assisted living, would be a reality for the individual diagnosed with dementia and family members.

The way forward

The CRPD is a useful tool for those committed to improving dementia-related policy and practice (Shakespeare et al, 2017). It has potential to offer legal protection (Article 12), service entitlement (Article 19), and can change the public's understanding of dementia (Article 8) (Mental Health Foundation, 2015). Now that dementia has been formally recognized by the ADI as a rights-based concern (Shakespeare et al, 2017), and representation has been made to the UN CRPD Committee by individuals living with dementia, there is a need for nations to collaborate more closely with the UN CRPD Committee in monitoring their countries' policy plans to ensure compliance. Likewise, the new global action plan on dementia (WHO, 2016), discussed in Chapter Three, which is heavily grounded in human rights principles, must be used by countries currently developing dementia strategies/plans and others updating their strategies. The global plan has been strongly influenced by the proceedings from the first global ministerial

conference on dementia (WHO, 2015b), along with written and informal feedback
received from 79 member states and other relevant key stakeholders.

So far this chapter has traced the key political events that have influenced public policy on dementia within Europe and globally. It has argued that the last decade has witnessed a proliferation of national dementia strategies, each committed to improving quality of care (Fortinsky and Downs, 2014) and quality of life for the individual living with dementia. Drawing on findings presented in earlier chapters, an argument was marshalled that a considerable gap exists between the objectives of policy plans and people's real-life experiences. One likely explanation for this is the limited involvement people living with dementia and their family members have traditionally had in dementia policy formulation and implementation. The chapter demonstrated that whilst the early national dementia strategies were underpinned by a biomedical understanding of dementia, more recent strategies tend to frame dementia as a public health (WHO, 2012), public health and human rights (WHO, 2016) and population health issue (Travers et al, 2015). It was argued that there are synergies between public policy on dementia and health promotion policies that have, to date, not been maximized. The next section of this chapter moves the debate forward to the important topic of the impact a rights–based approach has for practitioners working in the field of dementia care. But first, to a consideration of human rights awareness amongst practitioners.

Awareness of human rights and the implications of a rights-based approach for practitioners

Human rights are rights we all have and enjoy by virtue of being human. Whilst most of us are aware of our own rights, sometimes an awareness of the rights of others is not a top priority. For example, it is said that practitioners and policy-makers have a low level of awareness of the human rights of people living with dementia (Forbat, 2006). An understanding of rights is particularly important since, as argued in previous chapters, in terms of service provision, policy responses, funding allocation and research priorities, the individual and their family member may be significantly disadvantaged because of dementia. It is said that there is also a low awareness of human rights amongst older people themselves, healthcare staff and some academics (Kelly and Innes, 2012). Indeed, where human rights violations occur, it is noted that such incidents are seldom framed as human rights breaches or linked to broader 'societal and systemic processes...' (Kelly and Innes, 2012, p 65), but rather, can be interpreted as isolated one-off incidents. In this part of the chapter, attention turns to exploring the extent to which practitioners employed in care homes are aware of human rights standards in their daily work, and have witnessed incidents of the abuse of human rights in practice settings.

Chapter Three introduced the reader to the PANEL principles on human rights (WHO, 2015a) and the final part of this chapter will explore these principles from the perspective of practitioners and show that for staff who have received training in delivering person centred care, a rights-based approach to practice requires minimal new learning since the principles of human rights align well and extend on elements of person-centred care. But before progressing to that final discussion, attention is turned now to presenting the results from a recent Irish survey on human rights and dementia.

Survey of health service professionals and care staff

A survey on human rights was undertaken with a sample of practitioners attending three dementia training workshops held in Ireland in early 2017. Practitioners, all but three of whom had been working in the residential care sector, were asked to complete a self-administered questionnaire investigating their attitudes and views on human rights. Written and verbal consent was obtained for study participation. All those approached agreed to participate, and a total of 34 practitioners – 15 registered nurses, 12 healthcare assistants, two medical doctors and five others participated. Their mean age was 36 (the range was 25-61). Half had already undergone specialist training in dementia.

In response to a question asked, 'Have you up until today considered the human rights of people in your care?', about a quarter of the practitioners stated that they had not. Respondents were asked to provide examples of incidents they or their colleagues had observed where residents' rights had been breached, and half (N=17) could readily provide examples. Human rights abuses identified included the unethical use of physical restraints or AT/ST, as, for example, tying some residents to chairs with no documentation of such in care plans. One respondent reported she was encouraged to lie to a resident who required 'localization technology', and was advised to tell her that the wrist band which was used to set off an alarm was a blood pressure monitor. Other examples included residents being denied opportunities to pursue lifetime interests such as a priest being prevented from continuing to say mass in the nursing home lest he make mistakes, and in another case a resident who enjoyed listening to the radio no longer being permitted to do so.

Practitioners also cited examples of staff being rude to residents, not respecting their dignity and privacy rights, and some residents being denied the opportunity to partake in day trips or attend public ceremonies because of 'behaviours that challenge'. Other examples cited included residents being force fed, some not being allowed to exercise their retained abilities, and others being denied choice as, for example, not being allowed to get up or go to bed when they wanted. In one extreme case, a respondent said: "[They the residents are] treated very roughly, no consideration of privacy, [they are] naked on commodes, stripped naked at night to change bedclothes when wet. [They are] not washed before bed, [and] not cleaned after soiling. [They are] put to bed with false teeth in." She claimed that resources were so carefully rationed in the nursing home where she worked that no wipes were provided to clean residents who were incontinent. This meant that some staff supplied their own cleansing products. She also stated that during inspection times, the nursing home "put on a very good front". Referring to low staff-to-resident ratios, another respondent said, "[there is] not enough staff when needed, when residents need to go to the toilet and there is no one who might help them."

All but four practitioners surveyed reported that some form of AT/ST was used in the facility where they worked. Cameras reported on by 53 per cent of the respondents were the most common technology in use. These tended to be positioned in strategic areas, including dining rooms, corridors, day rooms, sitting rooms, main hall areas and outdoors. In a small number of cases no consent had been obtained from the residents for the use of such cameras. The second most common technology used and reported on by 11 practitioners were sensors linked to floor mats. Ten respondents reported that localization technology was used. In one-third of the nursing homes it was reported that some internal doors remained locked. Doors most likely to be locked included kitchens, medication rooms, staff offices, sluice rooms, dining rooms and storage rooms.

Finally, in response to a question asked, 'If you were aware that the rights of one of your residents was not being respected, would you report this?', all but two respondents stated that they would. Many practitioners were emphatic in their response here, making comments such as, "Yes, 100 per cent", "I'd do it immediately", and "yes, very definitely". In fact, several said that they had already reported similar incidents. In response to another question asked about possible barriers to whistleblowing, one-third could readily identify some barriers.

The most common barrier identified was 'fear of losing one's job'. A young male respondent new to the area said, "if pointed out, it may prompt a high investigation, then you could lose your job". An older female respondent reported, "sometimes it is easier to be silent about these things because they are requiring action and people do not want to deal with that."

A conclusion reached based on these findings is that the promotion of equality and human rights is not a reality for some individuals diagnosed with dementia who are resident in Irish nursing homes. Despite these findings and an awareness in some cases of the adverse consequences of whistle blowing, it is encouraging to note that the majority of practitioners claimed they would definitely report incidents of human rights violations were they to become aware of such. Findings point to the need for education and training on diversity, equality and human rights to be made compulsory for all health service professionals and care workers.

Health service professionals work within a professional code of ethics, and human rights values are closely allied to the values underpinning professional ethics. In social work, for example, respect for the inherent dignity and worth of persons, the pursuit of social justice, integrity of professional practice, confidentiality and competence in professional practice are all core professional values (CORU, 2011). Kinderman and Butler (2006, p 6) assert that the implementation of a rights-based approach in practice will be more effective if human rights are presented to workers as, 'complementary to well established value systems....' Apart from being closely aligned with professional values, human rights principles are also closely associated with elements of person–centred care, but a human rights framework goes a step further as it ensures best practice approaches are also in compliance with the law. In the final part of this chapter, I now return to exploring the PANEL principles introduced in Chapter Three, and demonstrate how these principles can be used by practitioners to interrogate practice, highlight inequities in dementia care and lobby for better resource allocation (Kelly and Innes, 2012).

Principles of a human rights-based approach and elements of person-centred care

In Chapter Three, the principles of a human rights-based approach for practice were introduced (see Table 3.2 in Chapter Three). These are the principles that ensure that the individual's fundamental freedom is respected, their autonomy is promoted and the person is treated with dignity and respect. The acronym 'PANEL' has been used to describe these principles, which reflect the core concepts of **p**articipation, **a**ccountability, **n**on-discrimination, **e**mpowerment and **l**egality (WHO, 2015a). These principles have also been adopted by the Scottish Government, in their *Charter of rights for people with dementia and their carers* (SPCPGA, 2009), and have been embedded in Scotland's second national dementia strategy (Scottish Government, 2013). These same five principles have been fully embraced by WHO (2015a), where it states:

> ... people living with dementia have the right to *participate* in society and ensure that those responsible for protecting the human rights of people living with dementia should be held *accountable* for any human rights violations. In addition there should be increased education about dementia to change attitudes of society and reduce stigma [*non-discrimination*]. Lastly people living with dementia should be *empowered* to participate in decision-making processes and to maintain their *legal* capacity. (WHO, 2015a, p 4; emphasis added)

Since the PANEL principles in my view are closely aligned with elements of person-centred care, the section that follows demonstrates the synergies between both. It is argued that a rights-based approach, when adopted by practitioners, offers a broad and solid framework for rigorous practice analysis and for anti-discriminatory work (Townsend, 2006). But first, to a brief overview of the concept of person-centred care.

Person centred care

To re-orientate the reader to elements of person-centred care, in this section I draw on Brooker and Latham's work (2016), and especially Brooker's earlier VIPS framework (2004), which was later embedded into the NICE/SCIE guidelines (2007). Brooker's analysis built on Kitwood's earlier works where the term 'person-centred care' was used by him to refer to non-medical care, which focused on the *person* and not the dementia and on care which revolved around the individual's interpersonal relationships and promoted wellbeing. The main task of dementia care, in Kitwood's view (1997b), was to maintain personhood (one's identity, selfhood and uniqueness), 'in the face of the failing of mental powers' (1997b, p 25). Kitwood (1993a) argued that much more could be done, beyond what was traditionally assumed, to sustain personhood, even in cases where people had a severe dementia. For Kitwood (1993a), best practice meant adopting the perspective of the individual, preserving their personhood, addressing their psychological needs and seeing the problem of dementia as being located both in the psychosocial environment as well as in the neurological impairment.

In extending Kitwood's theory on personhood and person-centred care, Brooker claimed that person-centred care (PCC) had four elements: a value base, an individualized approach, adopting the perspective of the individual, and providing a supportive social environment. Drawing on Kitwood's approach of using equations to communicate complex ideas, Brooker (2004) cleverly introduced a new equation, PCC=VIPS, where the acronym VIP is also used in English to describe **v**ery **i**mportant **p**eople. More recently Brooker and Latham (2016) have simplified these components as follows:

- 'V, a value base that asserts the absolute value of all human lives regardless of age or cognitive ability
- I, an individualized approach, recognizing uniqueness
- P, understanding the world from the perspective of the person identified as needing support
- S, providing a social environment that supports psychological needs.' (Brooker and Latham, 2016, p 12)

The VIPS framework is useful as it can easily be remembered and it recognizes how based on our humanity we are all valuable individuals who command dignity, autonomy and respect.

The PANEL principles

I now show how the PANEL principles (WHO, 2015a) are congruent with and build on elements of person-centred care identified by Brooker (2004). I also demonstrate how a rights-based approach to the training of health service professionals and other care staff can build on training underpinned by person-centred care philosophies.

Participation

The first of the PANEL principles is that of *participation*, and the topic of how people living with dementia can participate meaningfully in society has attracted much discussion over the years (see, for example, Marshall, 2005; Bartlett and O'Connor, 2007, 2010; Nedlund and

Nordh 2015). Less is known about how the active participation of an individual living with dementia can be denied when that person's information needs are not met (Rochford Brennan, 2016). We know, for instance, that many people who have dementia and their family members have significant information needs (Orrell et al, 2008; Begley, 2009; Diaz-Ponce, 2014). Examples include their need for information on:

- the diagnosis
- treatments (pharmacological and non-pharmacological)
- prognosis
- home adaptations/modifications including AT
- health and social care supports
- legal issues and
- financial management.

As shown in Chapter Four, if a person is not told they have dementia, they cannot own their diagnosis or consent to treatments and other post-diagnostic interventions. If a person and/or family member is not told about the availability of service providers such as dementia advisers/case managers, public health nurses, occupational therapists, social workers and so on then they cannot participate in decisions to access them. If at an early stage in the course of dementia a person is not advised about advanced planning tools such as enduring powers of attorney or advanced healthcare directives, they may be prevented from participating in important decisions likely to maximize their autonomy. If information about legal capacity is withheld, then the individual cannot insist on exercising choice and control in any decision-making. Knowledge and information are therefore the linchpin to ensuring continued meaningful participation. Treating people as individuals means giving them the necessary information required to enable them, along with a trusted family member, to make important decisions affecting their lives (Nuffield Council on Bioethics, 2009).

Table 6.1 reports on the synergies between elements of person-centred care as articulated by Brooker (2004), and a human rights-based approach to dementia care practice as espoused through the principle of participation. This principle of participation aligns well with that element of person centred care characterized as an individualized approach or in Brooker's own words, 'treating people as individuals' (Brooker, 2004, p 217). In terms of the Articles enshrined in the CRPD and discussed in preceding chapters, the principle of participation is particularly well embodied in Article 19 (independent living in the community), Article 25 (health), Article 26 (habilitation and rehabilitation) and Article 30 (participation in cultural life, recreation, leisure and sport). To help maximize the individual's active participation, practitioners can draw on the CRPD and use its Articles to cross-check whether those whom they support are being fairly treated and afforded equitable opportunities to participate in decisions that are directly relevant to their lives.

In applying this principle of participation to practice, the type of questions health service professionals and care staff need to consider include:

- Has the person living with dementia and other family members been given adequate information to enable them to actively participate in all decision-making affecting their lives?
- Has sufficient information been given to them about the diagnosis, its sub-type, their prognosis, drug treatments and other psychosocial interventions including cognitive stimulation therapy and cognitive rehabilitation?
- In viewing dementia as a disability, have any physical (including environmental), attitudinal or socio-political barriers been identified that might impede the full and effective participation of the individual and their family members in ordinary everyday life?
- If such barriers have been identified, how can they be eliminated?
- Has the person living with dementia and family members been given adequate information about home care services, peer support networks, dementia advisers, income supports including direct payments, AT, transport services, driving, advanced care planning tools and other legal supports?
- Has the person living with dementia and family members been given sufficient information about risk factors including information about exercise, diet, smoking, alcohol, blood pressure, social engagement, and so on?
- If the person can no longer live safely at home, has sufficient information been given to enable that person and family member to engage in decision-making about long-term care options?

Table 6.1: Human rights principles, elements of Brooker's person-centred care model and relevant Articles from the CRPD

Human rights PANEL principles	Brooker's elements of person-centred care	UN CRPD	Articles
Participation Everyone has the right to participate in decisions that affect their lives	Treating people as individuals	Living independently and being included in the community Health Habilitation and rehabilitation Participation in cultural life, recreation, leisure and sport	19, 25, 26, 30
Accountability Effective monitoring of human rights standards and remedies for breaches	A positive social environment in which the person living with dementia can experience relative wellbeing	General principles General obligations Awareness raising National implementation and monitoring	3, 4, 8, 33
Non-discrimination All forms of discrimination in the realization of rights are prohibited, prevented and eliminated with priority given to the most vulnerable	Valuing people with dementia and those who care for them	General principles General obligations Equality/non-discrimination Accessibility Equal recognition before the law Freedom from torture or cruel, inhuman or degrading treatment or punishment Living independently and being included in the community Respect for privacy	3, 4, 5, 9,12,15, 19, 22
Empowerment Individuals and communities should understand their rights and be supported to participate in the development of policy and practices that affect their lives	Looking at the world from the perspective of the person with dementia	General principles Equality and non-discrimination Equal recognition before the law Living independently and being included in the community	3, 5, 12, 19
Legality Recognition of rights as legally enforceable entitlements (linked to national and international law)	A positive social environment in which the person with dementia can experience relative wellbeing	General principles General obligations Accessibility Equal recognition before the law National implementation and monitoring	3, 4, 9, 12, 33

Accountability

Accountability is the second key principle in the PANEL or human rights-based approach to practice. WHO (2015a, p 2) notes that, 'Public and private bodies, non-governmental organizations and individuals who are responsible for the care and treatment of people with dementia should be held accountable for the respect and protection of their care recipients and adequate steps should be adopted to ensure this is the case.' For accountability to be effective, appropriate laws, policies and procedures must be in place to ensure human rights are upheld (SHRC, 2015), and practitioners need to be familiar with such legislation and know the appropriate mechanisms for redress when human rights are neglected or violated.

Accountability is paramount in all aspects of our personal and professional lives. It is particularly important for staff employed in human service organizations where the organization's 'raw materials' are often vulnerable people/clients (Jones and May, 1996) including service recipients, hospital patients or nursing home residents. Often practitioners tend to be aware of their accountability to organizational and professional bodies (Jones and May, 1996), including supervisors, co-workers, management boards, inspection authorities and professional associations, but they may be less well aware of their need to be accountable to those responsible for human rights legislation.

Table 6.1 reports on the synergies between that element of person-centred care, 'a positive social environment in which the person living with dementia can experience relative wellbeing' as articulated by Brooker (2004, p 216), and a human rights-based approach to dementia care practice as espoused through the principle of accountability. This principle is also embodied in several of the Articles already discussed in this book including Article 3 (general principles), Article 4 (general obligations), Article 8 (awareness raising in this context of dementia as a disability) and Article 33 (national implementation and monitoring). For practitioners working in the field these Articles can be drawn on to help ensure that the rights of those for whom they support are being respected and fulfilled. Likewise practitioners can use human rights legislation to protect their own rights. In approaching practice from a rights-based perspective and in the context of accountability, the type of questions health service professionals and dementia care staff need to consider include:

- Do I know who to consult should I have concerns about human rights breaches?
- What mechanisms of redress can I draw on to uphold the human rights of those I support?
- Am I familiar with my own country's legislation on human rights including equality acts, anti-discrimination acts, disability acts, mental health capacity/assisted decision-making capacity acts and any other relevant legislation?
- Am I familiar with my own country's public policy on dementia?
- Have I been given the opportunity to undergo training in human rights and dementia?
- If training in human rights is not available, who can I approach to organize this?
- If fearful of whistleblowing within my own human service organization, is there any Ombudsman, inspectorate or external organization I can report my concerns to?
- Are human rights considerations incorporated into the human service organization's promotional brochures and manuals?
- Are inspection procedures using the legal aspects of human rights requirements to ensure staff are being trained in human rights?
- Have care providers, including nursing home proprietors, provided the optimum conditions required to enable staff to practice within a human rights framework?

Non-discrimination

Non-discrimination, the third component of the PANEL principles, is an important aspect of all human rights treaties, and forms the bedrock of the CRPD. It means that all types of discrimination, direct and indirect, must be prevented and eliminated, with due priority given to those who are the most vulnerable (WHO, 2015a). Earlier chapters showed how because of dementia, an individual can be stigmatized and not treated on an equal basis with others. For example, a person may not have had the opportunity to obtain a diagnosis, receive treatments, participate in rehabilitation, avail of home care supports, enjoy a good quality of life and so on. At a personal level, discrimination can relegate the individual to the status of less than human (Kitwood, 1997a), but at a societal level it can lead to neglect and the deprivation of dignity and human rights (UNECE, 2015b). Woods (2001) asserts that discrimination at any level complicates the neurological impairment and reduces opportunities for development and growth.

The principle of non-discrimination (see Table 6.1) aligns well with that element of person-centred care, characterized as 'Valuing people with dementia and those who care for them' (Brooker, 2004, p 216). However, it extends beyond this, since an awareness of discriminatory practice can result in redress through legal frameworks including drawing on equality legislation. If people are valued regardless of their level of cognitive impairment (Nuffield Council on Bioethics, 2009), and if their personhood is promoted (Kitwood, 1997a), then it is unlikely they will be discriminated against. In relation to the CRPD, the principle of non-discrimination is well embodied in Articles 3 and 4 (general principles and general obligations), Articles 5 and 12 (equality and non-discrimination and equal recognition before the law) Article 9 (accessibility) and in Articles 15, 19 and 22 (freedom from torture or cruel, inhuman or degrading treatment and punishment, living independently and being included in the community and the right to privacy).

In the context of anti-discriminatory practice, the type of questions health service professionals and dementia care staff should ask include:

- Are people living with dementia being given the same opportunities as others to access mainstream health and social care supports irrespective of the severity of their cognitive impairment?
- What, if anything, is being done to promote the independence, autonomy, wellbeing and participation in decision-making for the person with dementia?
- Is the individual diagnosed with dementia being offered the same choices and opportunities to exercise control as those who are cognitively intact?
- In care homes, are the physical health needs of residents who have a cognitive impairment receiving the same medical attention, including referrals to specialist services, as those residents who do not have dementia?
- Have exceptionally vulnerable individuals been identified including the person with young onset dementia, the individual who lives alone, and the person whose dementia is significantly complicated because of co-morbidities and/or sensory impairment?

Empowerment

Empowerment is the fourth of the PANEL principles, and in the context of human rights, it refers to people knowing and understanding their rights and being able to claim them. Drawing on Parsons and Cox's work (1994), Bartlett and O'Connor (2010) argue that empowerment-focused practice requires consideration of the personal, interpersonal, environmental and political aspects of the problem at hand. Brooker and Latham (2016) maintain that empowering people requires an organizational culture that also empowers frontline staff to be responsible for everyday decision-making.

Table 6.1 shows how the principle of empowerment is congruent with element three of Brooker's VIPS framework (Brooker, 2004, p 216) namely, 'looking at the world from the perspective of the person with dementia'. In the context of the CRPD, and the human rights issues discussed in this book, the principles of empowerment are embodied in Article 3 (general principles), Article 5 (equality), Article 12 (equal recognition before the law) and Article 19 (living independently and being included in the community).

In approaching practice from a rights-based perspective and in the context of empowerment, the questions health service professionals and care staff need to ask here include:

- Are the views of people living with dementia and their family members central in key decision-making processes?
- Are people living with dementia and their families aware of their rights, and aware of how to claim their rights?
- If unable to self-advocate, who, if anyone, can adopt an advocacy role on the individual's behalf?
- Are there mechanisms in place in the local community such as Alzheimer societies, dementia-friendly communities and Alzheimer cafes to support the interdependence of people living with dementia with others?
- Are people living with dementia and their family members aware of these services and how to access them?
- If language skills are impaired, what alternate communication techniques can be used that might help capture that person's voice?

Legality

The final element of the PANEL principles and a human rights-based approach to practice is legality. Human rights are legally enforceable entitlements linked to national and international human rights legislation. WHO (2015a) asserts that in the context of dementia, all measures (policy, practice and research) adopted by countries globally should be linked to human rights standards embedded in legislation and in human rights instruments. A service may engage in aspects of good practice or person-centred care, but without an explicit human rights-based culture, including a working understanding of human rights legislation, it may not necessarily be rights-based (SHRC, 2015).

Table 6.1 shows that this principle of *legality* aligns well with that element of person-centred care, described as the provision of 'a positive social environment in which the person living with dementia can experience relative wellbeing' (Brooker, 2004, p 216). In the context of the CRPD, and those human rights topics discussed in previous chapters, the principle is embodied in Articles 3 and 4 (general principles and general obligations), Article 9 (accessibility) Article 12 (equal recognition before the law) and Article 33 (national implementation and monitoring).

In approaching practice from a rights-based perspective the type of questions health service professionals and dementia care staff need to consider here include:

- Does the country's national dementia strategy comply with human rights legislation and with treaties, especially the CRPD?
- If not, what aspects of policy need to be updated or changed to ensure compliance?
- Is the person with dementia recognized equally before the law?
- Have legal frameworks as, for example, mental health capacity acts, been amended/adapted to take account of legal capacity?
- Is legislation in place for supportive decision-making that respects legal capacity?
- Has all discriminatory legislation been abolished and replaced with legislation that ensures free and informed consent to interventions?
- In countries where the CRPD has been ratified, are people with dementia or their representatives involved in monitoring their countries' performance?

So far I have argued that a human rights-based approach to practice is congruent with and extends on elements of person-centred care (Brooker, 2004), since for practitioners, a rights-based framework ensures not only better work performance but it is a legal requirement (Kinderman and Butler, 2006). Human rights principles are also consistent with most people's fundamental values, complement professional codes of ethics and are said to consolidate principles widely shared by civil society (Kinderman and Butler, 2006). Under human rights acts, human service organizations have a legal responsibility to provide equitable services that demonstrate fairness and respect for the dignity and humanity of the individual. Healthcare professionals and care workers need to be aware of policies and legislation and know how to apply them in daily practice.

Kidd (2012, p 91) notes that human rights are embedded in empathy and understanding, and in 'a willingness to walk a mile in another person's shoes'. In this way a human rights perspective builds on elements of person–centred care by providing practitioners with a stronger moral and legal framework to work within. Human rights training does not necessarily require any change in ideology, but rather, training can complement fundamental views about fairness and equity (Kinderman and Butler, 2006). Like training to deliver person-centred care, training in human rights also needs to target both attitudes and knowledge (Redman et al, 2012), and a rights-based culture needs to be fully embedded in the entire organizational cultural environment (Audit Commission, 2003). With appropriate training, practitioners can use human rights legislation to tackle problems, improve services, obtain additional resources and empower other staff (Kelly and Innes, 2012). Since a concern about human rights should be at the very core of all interactions health service professionals and care staff have with people living with dementia and their families, training on human rights should be mandatory, regular and built into all courses, at both an undergraduate and postgraduate level.

Conclusion

This chapter has traced the development of public policy on dementia over the last decade. It has shown that in recent years a rights-based discourse is gradually beginning to gain traction in some countries' policy plans. However, it was argued that where reference to human rights occurs in policy plans, the emphasis is on civil and political rights and not on social and economic rights. This is not all that surprising since social and economic rights otherwise known as positive rights (see Chapter One) are resource-intensive (Quinn, 2009). The chapter has argued that there is a need for public policy on dementia to be reframed and transported from deficits-based models of support to rights-based models that position the individual at the fore and place a stronger emphasis on strengths, rights, assets and choice.

The second part of the chapter presented new findings on human rights and dementia collected from a sample of health service professionals and care staff. The data show that an awareness of human rights is not always high on the agenda of some Irish practitioners, and there is a need for training on human rights and for staff to apply human rights knowledge to enable them to interrogate and reframe their practice. Picking up on this theme, the final part of this chapter has attempted to operationalize human rights principles in ways that may be useful for practitioners. It is argued that human rights training can build on elements of person–centred care, but a human rights approach provides a more robust framework as it offers the potential for legal protection, service entitlement and a positive shift in the way in which dementia is conceptualized. Once familiar with the appropriate legislation (including mental health, disability, discrimination and human rights), and with basic human rights instruments including the CRPD, this approach can be used by practitioners to promote a better quality of life for all those whom they support (Kelly and Innes, 2012).

Summary of key points
- Many countries today have developed their own policy plans/national dementia strategies to address the challenge of dementia.
- Whilst earlier dementia strategies tended to be underpinned by a biomedical framing of dementia, more recent strategies reflect a broader biopsychosocial and public health perspective.
- A recent theme cross-cutting several of the newly evolving or updated national dementia strategies is that of human rights.
- This human rights emphasis in dementia strategies focuses on the promotion of negative rights such as respect, dignity, autonomy, self-determination and safety, and not on positive rights such as the right to welfare benefits and service supports.
- Traditionally, the individual living with dementia and their family members had very limited involvement in dementia policy formulation or implementation
- Policy-making is highly political, user engagement may be tokenistic and the user's voice, may be suppressed and far from equal with that of the voice of more powerful interest groups/ stakeholders.
- There is a need for more extensive non-tokenistic user engagement in the development of public policy on dementia, to ensure that policies are directly relevant to peoples' everyday lives and reflect their wishes and preferences.
- The CRPD and WHO's global action plan on the public health response to dementia are powerful tools that can be used to help to re-frame dementia policy.
- Awareness of human rights issues is only fair among health service professionals and care workers employed in some residential care settings in Ireland.
- Care home organizers have an obligation to ensure optimum conditions to enable staff practice within a human rights framework.

- Inspection authorities need to use human rights legislation to ensure that care homes provide the necessary conditions such as training, resources and leadership, to enable staff practice within a human rights framework
- A human rights-based approach to practice using the PANEL principles builds on and extends on elements of person-centred care.
- Health service professionals and care staff can use a human rights approach to enhance practice, improve services, obtain additional resources, improve communication and empower other staff.

Notes

[1] 'Legacy event' was the term given to conferences and other such events that occurred immediately following the G8 summit (2013), including some that took place in London, Canada, France, Japan and Washington (DH, 2015). Here I use the term broadly to refer to what constitutes, in my view, important milestones in the evolution of dementia policy.

[2] ADI define 'plans' as government-led actions in which the government holds itself accountable to measurable objectives, whilst 'strategies' are collaborative partnerships, usually between governments, NGOs and the health and social care sectors working together (see www.alz.co.uk/alzheimer-plans). Here I refer to strategies/plans interchangeably.

[3] The fourth French plan on dementia is part of the *French Plan Maladies Neuro-Degeneratives (2014-2019)*.

[4] Risk reduction messages for other chronic illnesses such as coronary heart disease and stroke are the same as for dementia, and yet in most countries synergies between these programmes have not, to date, been promoted.

SEVEN

Legal capacity for people with dementia: a human rights approach

Eilionóir Flynn[1]

Introduction

In this chapter I explore the right to legal capacity for people with dementia as set out in Article 12 of the UN CRPD. As has been demonstrated in earlier chapters in this volume (see Chapters Two and Three in particular), people with dementia come within the CRPD's conceptualisation of persons with disabilities, and therefore have access to all the rights contained in the Convention. My analysis in this chapter first focuses on General Comment No 1 of the UN CRPD Committee (OHCHR, 2014), which represents an authoritative interpretation of the treaty text by its monitoring body, and provides the clearest guidance to States Parties to the CRPD to date on how the right to legal capacity for persons with disabilities, including people with dementia, may be ensured.

Second, I provide some examples of law reform around the world on the issue of legal capacity, and consider how these proposed reforms might impact on people with dementia. In particular, I focus on the early reform efforts in the Canadian province of British Columbia (which occurred prior to the entry into force of the CRPD), and the most recent development at the time of writing, in the Republic of Ireland.

Finally, I consider how the right to legal capacity might be framed in any new UN Convention on the Rights of Older Persons, based on the discussions to date in the UN Open-Ended Working Group on Ageing. This analysis provides important insights into how the right to legal capacity might further evolve in international human rights law with the advent of a new treaty on the rights of older persons.

Article 12 of the CRPD and General Comment No 1

Some preliminary reference was made to Article 12 in Chapter Four of this volume, which examined the individual's right to a diagnosis, its disclosure and to live independently in the community. The right to legal capacity of persons with disabilities is expressed in Article 12 as a component of the right to equal recognition before the law. In essence, the right to legal capacity means the recognition of the individual as a person before the law, and as an actor before the law with legal rights and responsibilities. The CRPD draws on the approach of previous human rights conventions, such as Article 16 of the *International Covenant on Civil and Political Rights* (ICCPR), and the *Convention on the Elimination of All Forms of Discrimination Against Women* (CEDAW). In fact, it was through CEDAW that the term 'legal capacity' first appeared in international human rights law. Article 15 provided that 'States Parties shall accord to women, in civil matters, a legal capacity identical to that of men and the same opportunities to exercise that capacity. In particular, they shall give women equal rights to conclude contracts and to administer property....' The use of this term in the context of women demonstrates that 'legal capacity' means both the ability to hold rights, also referred to as legal standing, and the ability to exercise rights, for example, by entering contracts, also referred to as 'legal agency' (McSherry, 2012).

It is worth restating here for clarity that the text of the CRPD was negotiated with the active involvement of persons with disabilities and their representative organisations, including self-advocates with intellectual and psychosocial (mental health) disabilities. Their input directly shaped the final language of the Convention, including the text of Article 12. Further, the UN Committee that monitors the Convention is primarily composed of persons with disabilities – 17 of the 18 Committee members at the time of writing are persons with disabilities. Although there is no record of the direct involvement of people with dementia in negotiation of the text of the Convention, it is clear that the rights contained in the Convention were intended to apply to them.

Further, while some allies from organisations representing family members of persons with disabilities, such as Inclusion International, were actively involved in the drafting of the Convention, it is clear from the negotiation archive that the Convention text was developed from the perspective of persons with disabilities themselves, rather than from the perspective of family members. While family members are powerful allies in the global effort to recognise disability rights as human rights, their views and insights may differ from the perspective of those who have a lived experience of disability. This is also true in the context of dementia. Therefore, in understanding how the strong articulation of the right to legal capacity in Article 12 of the CRPD was arrived at, it is important to bear in mind the context in which this text was drafted with the significant input of people who had experienced denials of their rights to bodily autonomy, self-determination and decision-making, and sought to remedy this injustice through a clear and binding international human rights norm.

With the entry into force of Article 12, some innovative applications of the existing right to legal capacity emerged. The most important of these is the duty on States Parties in Article 12(3) 'to provide access by persons with disabilities to the support they may require in exercising their legal capacity.' This statement represents what Flynn and Arstein-Kerslake (2014) have referred to as the support model of legal capacity. Others, such as Browning, Bigby and Douglas (2014), refer to this as the recognition of supported decision-making in international human rights law. This represents a departure from what the UN CRPD Committee has referred to as 'substituted decision-making'. The text of Article 12 does not use the terms 'supported decision-making' or 'substituted decision-making'. These terms emerged when the UN CRPD Committee began to examine States Parties that had ratified the Convention, and provide guidance on the reforms still needed to ensure compliance with Article 12.

These terms were used by the Committee in its Concluding Observations on States Parties, but were not fully defined until the publication of General Comment No 1 in 2014. Unlike the text of the CRPD, the General Comment is not binding in international law; however, it represents an authoritative interpretation of the treaty text by its monitoring body. In international human rights law, States are only bound by the text of treaties at the time they ratified, and some have argued that the Committee has provided an interpretation of Article 12 that is different from the understanding States had of this Article at the time the CRPD negotiations concluded in 2006. However, other scholars have demonstrated that the Committee's approach is in keeping with the intentions of the drafters (including the representative organisations of persons with disabilities and many of the states involved in the negotiation process).

It is also worth noting that prior to the adoption of the General Comment, many States Parties and members of civil society had called for the Committee to clarify the meaning of supported decision-making and substituted decision-making, so that they could work towards reforming domestic laws, policies and practices. The fact that the Committee has produced this clarification with which some actors now disagree is to some extent irrelevant. Since the General Comment now represents the standard to which States will be held when they appear before the UN Committee, it is, in my view, advisable for all States to work towards compliance with its provisions, while remembering, as the Committee has stated, that no country that has been examined to date is as yet fully compliant with Article 12.

In the following section I discuss three important aspects of the General Comment that demonstrate how Article 12 can be applied in practice in domestic legal frameworks. The first is the definition of substituted decision-making and the requirement in the General Comment to abolish substituted decision-making regimes. The second is the distinction between mental capacity and legal capacity, already broadly touched on in Chapter Four of this volume, but which will be expanded on here, and the resulting critique of functional assessments of mental capacity where these are used to restrict or deny legal capacity. The final aspect is the definition of a supported decision-making regime, with examples of supports to exercise legal capacity that states must make available to persons with disabilities, including people with dementia.

Substituted decision-making

According to the UN Committee's General Comment, substituted decision-making involves removing the individual's legal right to make a particular decision, and vesting the authority to make that decision in a third party, who typically makes the decision in the perceived objective 'best interests' of the person (OHCHR, 2014). Substitute decision-makers can be state-appointed representatives or guardians, or family members or friends who take on this role. The Committee requires substituted decision-making regimes to be abolished and 'replaced with supported decision-making which respects the person's autonomy, will and preferences' (OHCHR, 2011). It is important to remember that not all delegations of decision-making responsibility violate this obligation to abolish substituted decision-making. As Arstein-Kerslake and Flynn have previously argued:

> There are some examples of the appointment of outside decision-makers which would not violate this … obligation set out in the General Comment. For example, where a person chooses to delegate decision-making on a particular

issue to a trusted person, whose role is to make the decision based on the appointer's will and preferences. This kind of delegation of decision-making responsibility should be available to persons with disabilities as well as persons without disabilities. (2016, p 477)

An obvious example of this approach in the context of dementia would be the use of advance planning tools, such as powers of attorney or advance directives. However, as will be explored further later, in order to comply with Article 12, the individual must have the discretion to determine when the appointment will take effect and on what conditions it can be terminated. Currently, these arrangements usually require the individual to demonstrate that she or he has mental capacity when making the appointment and the appointed person takes action on her or his behalf when someone else determines that the appointer has lost mental capacity. If we are to move beyond the capacity/incapacity paradigm as mandated by the UN Committee and discussed further later, then we must give greater flexibility to the appointer to determine when they want another person to act on their behalf and when they want to reclaim their own ability to act independently. This idea is discussed in further detail later.

During the drafting of the CRPD, there were lengthy debates about substituted decision-making and whether it could really be abolished for all people with disabilities – including those with the most significant and complex disabilities, such as people in the final stages of dementia. Discussions were held on the concept of 'one hundred per cent support', where a person with very high support needs would have their wishes interpreted for them by a supporter as an alternative to existing models of substituted decision-making (UN enable, 2006). Some, including the Chair of the Ad Hoc Committee, questioned whether this kind of intensive support was really distinct from substituted decision-making (UN enable, 2006). Since the adoption of the General Comment, it is now clear that the Committee requires the total abolition of substituted decision-making and its replacement with a wide range of options to support the exercise of legal capacity. As discussed further later, this does not mean that the Committee believes that all human beings possess the same decision-making abilities. Rather, the Committee recognizes the diversity of ability and support needs among people with disabilities, and requires States to acknowledge and support those who ask for assistance in exercising their right to legal capacity, rather than stripping them of the legal ability to make decisions for themselves.

Mental and legal capacity

The denial or restriction of legal capacity through substituted decision-making is often imposed as the result of an assessment that the individual lacks the 'mental capacity' necessary to make a particular decision. In this context, 'mental capacity' is used to refer to the decision-making skills or abilities of an individual. In the General Comment, the UN Committee has now made clear that in order to respect the individual's human rights, 'perceived or actual deficits in mental capacity must not be used as justification for denying legal capacity' (OHCHR, 2014, para 12). This approach reflects the commentary of scholars and activists who were actively involved in the negotiations of the CRPD. Dhanda (2006) describes how Article 12 presents humankind with two fundamental choices:

> One recognizes that all persons have legal capacity and the other contends that legal capacity is not a universal human attribute. To ask for the making of the first choice does not mean that it is also being contended that all human beings in fact possess similar capacities. Even as all human beings are being accorded similar value, the differences between them is not being ignored or devalued. The second, on the other hand, recognizes the fact that there are some human beings who do not possess legal capacity and hence can be declared incompetent. (2006, pp 457-8)

This perspective is important to consider when implementing the requirements of Article 12 as set out in the General Comment. It emphasizes that naturally, there are differences in the mental capacity or decision-making skills of individual human beings. However, it asks us to respond in a new way to these differences. Rather than seeing a person's decision-making skills as a deficit and removing the individual's right to make particular decisions as a result, we are asked to support that person to make the decision that accords with her or his will and preferences, within the boundaries of the law, as discussed in further detail later. This change in the understanding of capacity has very profound implications for people living with dementia.

In many countries, including Ireland and the UK, the current approach to assessments of mental capacity (and subsequent removals of legal capacity) is based on a functional test (Mental Capacity Act 2005). This test typically requires individuals to demonstrate that they can understand, retain, use and weigh information in order to make a decision, and communicate that decision to others, before their decision can be respected in law. The test often takes place in a clinical setting where the individual may feel ill at ease and disempowered. Where an individual is unable to complete one of these tasks in respect of a particular decision, she or he will be found to lack the mental capacity necessary to make that decision, and as consequence, her or his legal capacity to make that decision will be removed and vested in a third party – such as a decision-making representative, deputy or the court. The General Comment provides a strong critique of the use of functional assessments of mental capacity to deny legal capacity, stating:

> This functional approach is flawed for two key reasons. The first is that it is discriminatorily applied to people with disabilities. The second is that it presumes to be able to accurately assess the inner-workings of the human mind and to then deny a core human right – the right to equal recognition before the law – when an individual does not pass the assessment. In all these approaches, a person's disability and/or decision-making skills are taken as legitimate grounds for denying his or her legal capacity and lowering his or her status as a person before the law. Article 12 does not permit such discriminatory denial of legal capacity, but rather requires that support be provided in the exercise of legal capacity. (OHCHR, 2014, para 14)

Prior to the entry into force of the CRPD, and before the General Comment was published, many commentators, such as Appelbaum and Grisso (1995), argued that the functional assessment of mental capacity respected human rights norms. These authors further claimed that it was an improvement on previous approaches that denied legal capacity based on the individual's status (for example, as a person with a label of cognitive disability), or where the outcome of the individual's decision placed the person at risk of harm (a standard that still applies in laws that permit involuntary mental health treatment). However, as Dhanda (2006) and Flynn and Arstein-Kerslake (2014) have argued, the functional approach in practice does not provide any greater human rights protection than its predecessors – the status and outcome-based approaches.

In practice, functional assessments of mental capacity still discriminate against persons with disabilities, including those with a diagnosis of dementia. This is because these individuals are, on the basis of this diagnosis, far more likely to be required to undergo this assessment, and to have their legal capacity to make decisions restricted or denied as a result, than people without a diagnosis or disability (although non-disabled adults might be just as likely to have difficulty with making many of the same decisions). In light of this, the General Comment clearly states that:

> ... a person's status as a person with a disability or the existence of an impairment (including a physical or sensory impairment) must never be grounds for denying legal capacity or any of the rights provided for in article 12. All practices that in purpose or effect violate article 12 must be abolished in order to ensure that full legal capacity is restored to persons with disabilities on an equal basis with others. (OHCHR, 2014, para 9)

In legal systems where assessments of mental capacity are widespread (including Ireland and the UK), many have asked what would replace this assessment process if Article 12 is fully implemented. The answer is simple – a process to discover the will and preferences of the person (using the person's desired forms of support, where needed), which, once known, must be respected. This has very significant ramifications for people living with dementia, especially in terms of being afforded opportunities to engage in advance care planning. This idea is discussed further in the following section.

Moving from 'best interests' to 'will and preferences'

In order to achieve the paradigm shift of Article 12 of the CRPD, the General Comment asks States to abolish substituted decision-making regimes that use 'best interests' standards to impose decisions on persons with disabilities who are deemed to lack mental capacity. Instead, States must provide support for the exercise of legal capacity based on the individual's 'rights, will and preferences'. While the General Comment does not explain in more detail what is meant by the term 'will and preferences', Arstein-Kerslake and Flynn have argued that based on the Committee's jurisprudence, an individual's 'will' can be understood as that person's long-term vision for their life, whereas 'preferences' might refer to the individual's likes and dislikes, or how the person prioritises specific goals (2016, pp 483-4).

The General Comment acknowledges that in some situations a person's will and preferences may be unknown, even after significant efforts to discover the individual's wishes have been made by her or his supporters. This includes where a person is in a coma or is not communicating in ways that others can understand. The Committee asks that in these situations, once all efforts to discover the person's wishes have been made, supporters proceed on the basis of their 'best interpretation' of the person's will and preferences on the relevant decision. This approach will likely be guided by supporters' knowledge of that person's life history, decisions they have made in the past and their values and beliefs. Such techniques are particularly relevant for people with dementia and their supporters. However, where an individual has no natural supporters who could provide these insights into their will and preferences, external decision-makers will still have to take a 'best interpretation' approach, and in this case, will likely rely on some baseline assumptions, such as that human beings generally want to live, and want to be free of pain.

Again, some authors, such as Ward (2015), have argued that the best interpretation approach in situations of last resort is not that distinct from best interests tests. After all, some best interests approaches, such as that contained in the Mental Capacity Act of England and Wales, include consideration of the person's wishes, values and beliefs as a component of best interests determinations. However, there is a clear difference between considering wishes and feelings as part of an external evaluation of a person's 'best interests' and actually making a decision that, to the best of our knowledge, truly respects a person's will and preferences. The key difference, for example, in England and Wales, is that wishes must be considered, but do not need to be respected under the law. The best interpretation of 'will and preferences' clearly requires the person's wishes, where known, to be respected within the boundaries of the law.

Some argue that the use of the phrase 'rights, will and preferences' in Article 12(4) means that certain rights can trump an individual's will and preferences (Law Society of Scotland, 2013). So, for example, if an individual wishes to refuse treatment that may result in her or his death, some would argue that she or he should be forced to undergo treatment in order to preserve her or his life. In this example, the right to life would trump the individual's will and preferences to refuse treatment. However, reading the CRPD as a whole, such an approach is not permissible, because the right to health in Article 25 requires that all healthcare be provided based on 'informed consent'. No provision, therefore, is made in the CRPD for substituted decision-making or over-riding an individual's will and preferences in favour of some external decision-maker's view of what constitutes the person's 'rights'.

A more difficult question arises when the person's will and preferences are constantly changing or where the person has conflicting wishes. An example of this is where a person expresses a wish to live but refuses live-saving medical treatment. In these cases, careful deliberation of how conflicting wishes can be reconciled is required. Many of us hold conflicting views on a wide range of issues – for example, I might want to be fitter, but refuse to exercise. We all struggle to reconcile our conflicting wishes, and people with dementia are no different. Often, conflicting wishes can be reconciled with time, and where a decision in these circumstances can be delayed, this can provide the time needed to give the required support. The goal of a 'best interpretation' approach is to attempt to reconcile the person's will and preferences in order to reach a decision – even where it is incredibly challenging to achieve such a reconciliation.

In many of these situations the 'best guess' of a trusted and chosen supporter, based on all the knowledge gathered about the person's past and present wishes, hopes and aspirations for her life, values and beliefs, is the most that can be achieved. The value and distinctiveness of this approach, while difficult, is its focus on the person and its efforts to understand and respect their perspective, even when it seems radically different from choices a supporter might make in her or his own life. With these interpretations, the provisions of the General Comment still represent a radical shift from existing approaches to determining the person's 'best interests', and this is a shift that has begun to be reflected in various domestic law reform efforts that are discussed in more detail in the following.

Law reform: British Columbia and the Republic of Ireland

One of the most well-known examples of legislation that provides for supported decision-making is the Representation Agreement Act in British Columbia. While the Act was developed prior to the CRPD, it contains a number of elements that are broadly aligned with the support model of legal capacity articulated above. However, it should be noted that this legislative framework is not fully compliant with the interpretation of Article 12 provided in the General Comment, particularly since it does allow for representatives to make decisions on behalf of the person, which do not necessarily respect the person's will and preferences. As already stated above, no legal system is, at the time of writing, fully compliant with Article 12. However, since this is one of the most commonly cited legislative examples of supported decision-making, it deserves further exploration.

The process of developing a 'representation agreement' under British Columbian law is very similar to granting a power of attorney. In the process of developing this legislation, senior citizens were amongst the most powerful civil society actors who demanded the introduction of these agreements as an alternative to the existing system of adult guardianship. Given the potential of these agreements to be used later in life and/or when communication abilities may decline, the agreements are particularly relevant for people with dementia. A representation agreement can cover a wide range of decisions, from financial decisions, to medical treatment, healthcare and personal care. As long as an individual is not 'incapable of doing so' (Representation Agreement Act, 1996, section 4), she or he can enter into a representation agreement with a support person or network that is appointed to assist her or him with decision-making. One of the innovations in this Act was its flexible approach to determining capability for the purpose of entering an agreement. The goal of the drafters was to ensure that as many people as possible would be recognized as capable of making these agreements, in order to provide a meaningful alternative to adult guardianship and other forms of substituted decision-making (Stainton, 2005).

Although there are flaws in the representation agreement system, it has a number of progressive elements that deserve further attention. The broad approach to determining capability for making, revoking or changing an agreement is a particular strength of this model. In British Columbia, an adult who wishes to enter into a representation agreement does not need to demonstrate a high level of mental capacity to enter into the agreement, as would be required for other legally-binding agreements. The person need only communicate a desire to have a representative, be able to demonstrate choices and have a relationship of trust with the representative (1996, section 8(2)). Therefore, a person who requires a great deal of support, and may not be able to communicate in conventional ways, is allowed to enter into a representation agreement by demonstrating trust in one or more supporters (1996, section 12(1)).

The representation agreements in British Columbia also contain a well-developed system of protection against abuse. Each individual entering into a representation agreement has the option of appointing a monitor in addition to her or his representative. In cases in which the representation agreement concerns the management of the individual's financial affairs, the appointment of a monitor is obligatory (1996, section 12(1)). The British Columbian approach has provided inspiration and guidance for many other jurisdictions, including Ireland, which have subsequently introduced legal recognition for various forms of supported decision-making agreement.

Ireland developed its reform of legal capacity law after it signed the CRPD but prior to ratification as part of a process of bringing laws into conformity with the Convention. The Assisted Decision-Making (Capacity) Act 2015 introduces for the first time in Irish law formal mechanisms for support to exercise legal capacity that do not amount to substituted decision-making – namely, decision-making assistance agreements, co decision-making agreements and advance healthcare directives. However, it also provides for enduring powers of attorney and the court appointment of decision-making representatives, which are closer to the definition of substituted decision-making regimes provided in the General Comment, as discussed above. The key difference between these roles and the traditional forms of substituted decision-making is that the person appointed is not permitted to make decisions based on her or his perception of the 'best interests' of the person, but rather, must make decisions that respect the person's will and preferences, as far as practicable.

However, the Act also retains the functional assessment of mental capacity as a trigger for imposing a decision-making representative on a person, and denying the person's legal capacity to make the relevant decision independently. The Act states that a person lacks capacity if she or he is unable:

> (a) to understand the information relevant to the decision, (b) to retain that information long enough to make a voluntary choice, (c) to use or weigh that information as part of the process of making the decision, or (d) to communicate his or her decision (whether by talking, writing, using sign language, assistive technology, or any other means) or, if the implementation of the decision requires the act of a third party, to communicate by any means with that third party. (2015, section 3(2))

I now consider each of the key provisions of the Act in turn to determine how they might be used by people with dementia, and the extent to which they meet the General Comment's definition of 'support to exercise legal capacity' in Article 12.

The decision-making assistant's role is simply to support the appointer in accessing information, considering options, ascertaining the appointer's will and preferences, and ensuring that the person's decision is implemented. The Act is clear that 'a decision-making assistant shall not make a decision on behalf of the appointer' (2015, section 14(2)). In this way, the Irish Act is distinct from the Representation Agreement Act in British Columbia that does allow representatives appointed in an agreement to make decisions on behalf of the person. While the Act does not require the appointer to prove her or his mental capacity to enter into an agreement, it does state that the appointer must consider her or his capacity is 'in question or shortly may be in question' (2015, section 10(1)) in order to make an agreement. The Act also states that the Minister must make regulations concerning the creation of decision-making assistance agreements, which should provide for the inclusion in the agreement of a statement 'by the appointer, that he or she has read and understands the information as to the effect of making the appointment or that such information has been explained to the appointer, by a person other than the proposed decision-making assistant' (2015, section 10(4)(d)(i)). This is the most flexible option under the Act in which the appointer retains full legal capacity and one that will hopefully be of use to people with dementia. However, the existence of a decision-making assistance agreement does not prevent a court from subsequently finding that the person lacks mental capacity and appointing a decision-making representative, which is a concern for people with advanced dementia along with those who have other significant cognitive disabilities.

The co-decision-making agreement is a step up in the intensity of support as, unlike the assistance agreement, it grants the appointed person the power to make decisions jointly with the appointer. In keeping with this increase in legal powers to the co-decision-maker, this agreement is more formal, and requires the inclusion of a statement by a registered medical practitioner and another healthcare professional that:

> ... in their opinion –
>
> i) the appointer has capacity to make a decision to enter into the co decision-making agreement,
> ii) the appointer requires assistance in exercising his or her decision-making in respect of the relevant decisions contained in the co-decision-making agreement, and
> iii) the appointer has capacity to make the relevant decisions specified in the co decision-making agreement with the assistance of the co-decision-maker. (2015, section 21(f))

Co-decision-makers are, however, bound to respect the guiding principles of the Act, which means that in making decisions jointly, they must respect the wishes of the appointer regarding the decision to be made, 'unless it is reasonably foreseeable that such acquiescence … will result in serious harm to the appointer or to another person' (2015, section 25(b)).

The final option for support to exercise legal capacity under the Act is the advance healthcare directive. The person creating the directive must demonstrate that she or he has mental capacity at the time the directive is made, and the directive is activated when the person has lost mental capacity. Since this continues to reinforce the capacity/incapacity paradigm, it conflicts with the General Comment, and does not provide the desired flexibility for the person herself or himself to set the conditions under which she or he wishes the directive to be activated. These directives can be made concerning physical or mental healthcare decisions, although they will no longer be binding if the person who makes it is subsequently treated as an involuntary patient under the Mental Health Act. This discrepancy was severely criticized by mental health activists such as Morrissey (2015) during the debates on the Act, and the Minister made a commitment to reform the Mental Health Act to ensure that advance directives can be given more legal weight, even when the person is made an involuntary patient (Seanad Éireann, 2015). As part of the directive, the person can appoint a healthcare representative to ensure that the directive is carried out. It is also important to note here that a person can only make legally binding refusals of treatment in the directive and cannot make legally binding treatment requests.

The Act also provides for the creation of enduring powers of attorney to cover all kinds of decisions – regarding personal welfare, or property and affairs. Until the Act was passed, people could only make enduring powers of attorney in Ireland on financial matters, and did not have the option to grant broader powers of attorney. However, the donor of the power must demonstrate that she or he has mental capacity at the time the power is made, and the power comes into effect when a medical practitioner and another health professional certify that the person has now lost the mental capacity to take decisions independently. Finally, the person will be appointed a decision-making representative if the court deems that the person lacks mental capacity to make a relevant decision. Decision-making assistants, co decision-makers, healthcare representatives appointed in an advance directive and attorneys must all be people who are already known to the person and chosen by her or him. The decision-making representative chosen by the court could either be someone known to the person (such as a family member or friend), or could be an independent appointee selected from a panel that will be operated by the Decision Support Service, a new body within the Mental Health Commission, established to oversee the implementation of the Act. In situations where a person is deemed to lack mental capacity, the court also retains the power to make a decision directly on her or his behalf, without appointing a representative, where the decision is urgent or where the court considers it expedient to do so.

The person who is appointed a representative does not have a say in who that representative will be, and cannot refuse to accept the representative appointed by the court. Further, the appointment of the representative is made based on a determination by the court that the person lacks mental capacity, and this appointment restricts the exercise of that person's legal capacity in respect of the relevant decision. Therefore, the representative role contravenes the requirement in the General Comment that perceived or actual deficits in the person's mental capacity should never be used as justification for denial of legal capacity. However, the representative is still bound to respect the guiding principles of the Act, and cannot make decisions based on the perceived 'best interests' of the person, but rather, must make decisions that respect, as far as practicable, the will and preferences of the person.

For many people with dementia, the introduction of decision-making assistance agreements and advance healthcare directives is an important development that will enable them to continue to exercise legal capacity over key decisions in their lives, even at times where their communication has changed or cognitive skills have declined. However, the Assisted Decision-Making (Capacity) Act clearly does not go far enough to comply with the interpretation of Article 12 set out in the General Comment. There is also the risk that many people with dementia, who are not currently subject to substituted decision-making regimes in Ireland, will experience pressure to enter agreements, as third parties such as banks and healthcare professionals or service providers may refuse to transact with them unless an agreement is in place. Further, there is a significant risk for people with advanced dementia that decision-making representatives will be imposed on them against their wishes, if they are found to lack mental capacity by the court.

Future directions: the potential of a Convention on the Rights of Older Persons

Since the decision of the UN General Assembly (2010) to establish an Open-Ended Working Group on Ageing (OEWGA), the idea that the next international human rights treaty might be one on the rights of older people has gained ground. The resolution set out the purpose of the group as follows: 'strengthening the protection of the human rights of older persons by considering the existing international framework of the human rights of older persons and identifying possible gaps and how best to address them, including by considering, as appropriate, the feasibility of further instruments and measures.' Therefore, it seems open to the group to recommend the adoption of a new human rights treaty to specifically address the rights of older people. The resolution also provided for the active involvement of civil society in the work of the open-ended group, and many organisations representing people living with dementia, such as Dementia South Africa and ADI, have participated in the six sessions of the working group to date.

At the time of writing, no formal negotiation has commenced of a draft Convention on the Rights of Older Persons. Nevertheless, the issue of legal capacity has been subject to some discussion in the five sessions to date of the OWEGA. While many civil society organisations and speakers in the sessions have highlighted the importance of self-determination and autonomy for older persons, there seemed to be less resistance, at least in the early sessions, to the idea that the exercise of legal capacity will be limited for older people as they acquire disabilities such as dementia, when compared with the discussions on legal capacity that took place in the Ad Hoc Committee. Evidence of this is found in the discussions of regional developments such as draft Conventions, protocols and recommendations on the human rights of older persons at the OEWGA from Africa (African Union), the Americas (Permanent Council of the Organisation of American States) and Europe (Council of Europe). These documents have sometimes contained weaker protections of the right to legal capacity for older people when compared with the right as framed in Article 12 of the CRPD, discussed above.

Although the UN OEWGA is not currently negotiating a draft text of a Convention, civil society organisations have begun to formulate the elements they believe should be present in a legally binding human rights instrument. For example, a concrete proposal developed by HelpAge International states that older people should have 'legal capacity on an equal basis with others in all aspects of life' and the 'support required to exercise legal capacity and to be complete citizens and to be an equal member of the family and of society' (2015, p 4). Similarly, it states that older people have a right to 'autonomy, self-determination and choice in all aspects of older people's lives including in making decisions about their support and care and leisure time, property, income, finances, place of residence, health and medical treatment or care, and funeral arrangements' (2015, p 4). In the context of the right to health, this draft states that older persons should have 'autonomy in terms of informed consent for, and choice of, treatment' and the 'opportunity to make advance instructions about health care, including palliative and end of life care' (2015, p 7).

These examples demonstrate the opportunities and challenges facing the drafting of a new Convention in terms of the framing of a right to legal capacity for older persons. On the one hand, based on discussions to date, there is a risk that this right will be framed more restrictively for older persons than it currently is for persons with disabilities – as evidenced by the regional developments discussed above. However, on the other hand, there is a real opportunity to expand the existing right to legal capacity for persons with disabilities to all older persons, and also to reconceptualize how this right can be framed positively in the context of making advance decisions – something that was not fully addressed in the CRPD. New interpretations of this right for older persons could, in turn, influence the development of new ideas in the disability movement on the recognition and protection of legal capacity for all.

Conclusion

In light of these recent developments, it is clear that legal capacity is a critical human rights issue in the context of dementia. Article 12 of the CRPD and General Comment No 1 provide a strong base for respecting the autonomy and self-determination of people with dementia, and recent law reform developments around the world are increasingly recognizing the need for support to exercise legal capacity. The 'will and preference' paradigm is gaining ground over the more paternalistic approach based on objective 'best interests' – and this has significant consequences for people with dementia who desire support to exercise legal capacity. Nevertheless, it has proved difficult in many law reform efforts to fully displace the functional assessment of mental capacity, which remains a trigger for the imposition of substituted decision-making and denials of legal capacity.

At the global level, the prospect of a new human rights treaty for older people might be well-placed to develop creative solutions in order to respect autonomy while providing appropriate support, and clarifying how will and preferences might be interpreted in the 'hard cases' where the person's wishes are unknown. Indeed, the opportunities for developing ideas on legal capacity for people with dementia within the UN OEWGA may well give rise to Jennings' conception of 'memoralized personhood'. He argues that:

... [t]o be a memorial person is to be a self in the imagination and memory of others; which on this view, is just what it is to be a self. It is to be a self whose identity and life must be honored and acknowledged by those who can, even if it can no longer be by the person himself or herself. And to be a self of any type – including a memorial person – is to be a self to whom, as Arthur Miller puts it in Death of a Salesman, "attention must be paid". (Jennings, 2010, p 176)

In order to ensure that we pay attention to the will and preferences of people with dementia, a robust conceptualization of legal capacity, which acknowledges the diversity of the human population and the different factors that influence our decision-making, is certainly required.

Summary of key points
- The human rights of people with dementia are protected by the CRPD.
- Article 12 of the CRPD protects the equal right to enjoy and exercise legal capacity.
- The right to legal capacity, according to the UN Convention, cannot be restricted or denied based on perceived or actual mental capacity.
- People with dementia who wish to use support to exercise their legal capacity should be facilitated to do so, and this support should be legally recognized.
- Advance planning, including the creation of living wills, advance directives or powers of attorney, can, if properly framed, be considered supports for people with dementia to exercise legal capacity. Some countries, including Ireland and Canada, have already passed laws to recognize supported decision-making mechanisms that could be used by people with dementia.

Note
[1] Eilionóir Flynn is a Senior Lecturer at the School of Law and Director of the Centre for Disability Law and Policy, National University of Ireland Galway.

EIGHT

Conclusions: grounds for hope

Across the world about 47 million people are estimated to have dementia and this figure is likely to rise to 131 million by 2050 (Winblad et al, 2016). The magnitude of dementia therefore cannot be ignored and the condition touches each of us in different ways and few will escape its reach. For dementia is not simply about the mind, the brain, memory loss and a decline in cognitive and functioning skills: it is also about personhood, selfhood and about who and how we are as human beings (Sabat, 2001), in a world where intact memories tend to be overvalued, and where an unprecedented emphasis is placed on rationality, thinking, cognitive competencies and economic productivity (Hughes, 2014).

In this way, dementia represents both a decline from a previous mental state and a very significant disconnect from the mainstream values of the dominant culture (Post, 2000). The fear and stigma of dementia is such that when talking about his diagnosis, the late Sir Terry Pratchett commented, 'It occurred to me that at one point it was like I had two diseases – one was Alzheimer's and the other was knowing I had Alzheimer's' (quoted in Alzheimer's Society, 2008, p ix). Thinking about dementia requires a willingness to take on board different perspectives (Innes, 2009) and an awareness of the different contributions disciplines such as biology, politics, biomedicine, economics, sociology, social policy, ethics and philosophy can make. Dementia is everyone's fascination yet sadly nobody's core responsibility.

The aim of this book has been to challenge conventional thinking about dementia, to introduce a fresh conceptual lens and provide new analytical tools to interrogate policy and practice in order to promote the individual and their family members' quality of life. I have also tried to bring the reader closer to the real life experiences of the individual who has the condition by citing their words in order to highlight some of the injustices and discrimination experienced. Reframing dementia as a rights-based issue is not new; however, what I have attempted to do is provide a more rigorous analysis of dementia-related practice and policy in order to demonstrate how a rights-based framework can offer new hope and provide a catalyst for social change.

Human rights are potentially powerful levers for social and political change (McGettrick, 2014), and denying a person their human rights is said to be equivalent to challenging their humanity (Mandela,

1990). Throughout this book I have shown how a person living with dementia is likely to encounter a wide range of social and structural barriers which can create additional disabilities and which can threaten their human rights. Because of this, there is need for greater awareness of dementia and human rights, for significant policy reform and for rights-based approaches to be incorporated into dementia policy and practice (Mental Health Foundation, 2015). A key recommendation is that policy-makers need to be more cognizant of human rights – social, economic and cultural along with civil and political rights. Another key recommendation is that practitioners need to undergo training in dementia and human rights and use a human rights framework in their everyday practice.

Opening the debate: a new conversation

For most of the 20th century, dementia in older people was seen as senility and an expected (normal) aspect of the ageing process. It was not until 1968 that Blessed et al demonstrated that at post-mortem the brains of older people who died with 'senile dementia' had the same neuropathological features of Alzheimer's disease, until then seen as a neurodegenerative condition only affecting younger people. This led to a disease and pathology model of dementia, which continues to predominate in the search for a cure and disease modifying treatments (Innes and Manthorpe, 2013). However, more recently the contributions of social scientists have provided alternative frameworks such as personhood (Kitwood, 1997), selfhood (Sabat, 2001), social citizenship (Bartlett and O'Connor, 2010) and human rights (Kelly and Innes, 2012). In this book a rights based framework has been applied to help to theorize the social and political aspects of dementia.

Since human rights is often considered a complex topic, in applying the human rights lens to dementia, I have deliberately kept my theorizing straightforward. For example, thresholds for the satisfaction and non-satisfaction of human rights have been introduced in a simplistic, binary way, when I know that these thresholds vary enormously: from at one extreme, the most adequate fulfilment of rights, to at the other, a total lack of fulfilment and violation of human rights (Townsend, 2006). Likewise, the pure social model of disability, which overlooks the biological determinants of disability such as 'impairment' (UPIAS 1976), and instead focuses exclusively on social determinants, has limitations when applied to dementia: the person living with dementia has both an impairment (neurological) along with disabilities (inabilities), both of which limit activities and restrict participation in society.

I am also conscious that just as the 'biomedical lens' cannot embrace the subjective experience of dementia, nor the 'personhood lens' the nuances of power relations in society, nor the 'citizenship lens' the complexities of human experience, (Bartlett and O'Connor, 2010), neither can the 'human rights lens' ignore the need for good clinical care and for biomedical research to proceed, which will hopefully one day find a cure. All perspectives have their limitations, and the goal should be to adopt a holistic approach, neither favouring one perspective over another (Bartlett and O'Connor, 2010), but rather, distilling from each, those insights that may help to expand thinking, and ensure that the person living with dementia and their family members are treated fairly and can enjoy a good quality of life.

In this concluding chapter, I draw together the dominant themes that underpin the book and highlight some of the core take-home messages that policy-makers, practitioners and researchers might bring forward. The discussion is centred on two broad topics, namely, 'grounds for hope' and 'a life of quality and equality'.

Grounds for hope

Strong leadership: the role of ADI and WHO

The multiple challenges dementia poses point to the need for strong political leadership of dementia at a global level, and despite the many examples of human rights breaches discussed in this book, I believe there are now clear grounds for hope. This statement is based on the fact that today there is evidence of firm political and global leadership of dementia, as seen in the joint collaborations recently forged between the ADI and WHO.

For many years the ADI has been successful in raising professional and public awareness of dementia and influencing policy through its high-quality research agenda. However, it is only since 2012, and probably as a result of the solid evidence base its scientific programme has consistently generated, that WHO has entered into partnership with the ADI to produce the report, *Dementia: A public health priority* (WHO, 2012). That report has been critical in reframing dementia as a public health issue, and providing the initial knowledge base required for governments, policy-makers and other stakeholders globally, to equip themselves for the challenge of dementia. WHO and the ADI's partnership, their firm commitment to reduce the impact of dementia and their appeal to all stakeholders to ensure that health and social care systems across the world become responsive to the challenge of dementia (WHO, 2012) augurs much hope for the future.

The new and strong leadership role adopted by WHO and the ADI is also reflected in their organizing, in 2015, the world's first ministerial conference on global action against dementia (see Chapter One). That global conference attended by representatives from 89 countries from around the world, including a large group of government ministers, has helped to further prioritize dementia as a global health issue. It has also helped to place the human rights framing of dementia on to the political agenda, and has acted as a springboard for WHO's Executive Council to request a global action plan on dementia (Rees, 2017).

Action areas

The resultant global action plan (WHO, 2016) discussed in Chapter Three (see final part) demonstrates a clear vision and sets an achievable agenda for dementia policy development worldwide over the next eight years (2017-25). Developing this policy plan involved an impressive consultative process, with WHO's member states, along with UN organizations and non-state actors, all actively involved in its drafting and development. It reflects global solidarity in dementia initiatives and a readiness for joint action. The global action plan prioritizes seven key policy areas namely:

- Dementia as a public health priority
- Dementia awareness and friendliness
- Dementia risk reduction
- Dementia diagnosis treatment care and support
- Support for dementia carers
- Information systems for dementia
- Dementia research and innovation

Most importantly, WHO will adopt an active role in addressing some of the action areas as, for example, through its development of e-health tools for caregivers and through its development of a global dementia observatory (Rees, 2017). All of these activities reflect strong political leadership and a commitment on the part of WHO to reduce the impact of dementia. This type of leadership and global solidarity is so important, as all of us are at risk of developing dementia, and together we must collectively take action and recognize that we all have responsibility to support the individual coping with the symptoms and their family members (Nuffield Council on Bioethics, 2009).

Newly emerging dialogues in dementia

A second indicator of why the future looks promising is reflected in how the dominant discourse on dementia is now being strongly challenged by the powerful voices of self-advocates. The recent legitimizing of the 'collective voice' as evidenced in the DAI developing a 'memorandum of agreement' with the ADI (Glenn Rees, personal communication, 2016) augurs further hope and will undoubtedly generate a more measured and compelling future debate since as noted by McGettrick (2014), 'nobody can deny the authoritative voice of the lived experience.' In their adopting the slogan borrowed from disability activists, 'nothing about us without us', both individually and collectively (through organizations like the DAI, dementia working groups along with others), the voice of people living with dementia has been successful in highlighting the type of social injustices experienced.

Through the ongoing exemplary effort of individuals like Kate Swaffer, Professor Peter Mittler, Christine Bryden, Helen Rochford Brennan, Ronan Smith, Kathy Ryan and Anne Johnson (along with many others around the world), their written and oral narratives have helped to level the playing field and weaken the dominant discourse. The DAI has led the campaign for access to the CRPD: it has influenced the ADI's decision to adopt a human rights-based policy that includes using the CRPD in policy development, and has submitted its own report to the UN CRPD Committee (Shakespeare et al, 2017).

Whilst their voice has been most persuasive in highlighting issues such as discriminatory practices and policies, and the need for dementia to be recognized as a disability, challenging the dominance of the biomedical model has not, as yet been included in their campaign. For example, some of the easy, cheap, quick-fix solutions referred to in earlier chapters in this book, and used in some care settings without any consideration given to the adverse consequences these solutions have on the human rights of the individual, have not yet been fully taken on board by them. Obviously self-advocates cannot do everything and challenging such policies, including the excessive or inappropriate use of antipsychotic medication, will take courage (O'Sullivan, 2013) but these are also important rights-based issues that need to be prioritized in future advocacy work.

Reframing the policy agenda

A third indicator of why the future looks promising for people living with dementia is reflected in the new global action plan on dementia (WHO, 2016) since as stated earlier, the plan which explicitly refers to the CRPD, is firmly embedded in human rights principles and highlights the need for countries to ensure that their policies and legislation comply with CRPD Articles. The plan also requires countries to submit regular reports to WHO outlining their progress in relation to policy development. Although countries are not legally required to meet the targets identified, a monitoring system will be put in place, whereby the ADI will be proactive in ensuring that member countries remain accountable to WHO (Mark Wortmann, personal communication, 2017). WHO has also agreed to provide technical advice to countries developing or revising their policy plans. These top-down initiatives are laudable, but what is needed to support such approaches is concerted action on the part of all stakeholders to help build a society that is more inclusive and supportive of the individual who has dementia and that person's family members.

The life course approach embedded in WHO's public health response to dementia (WHO, 2016) where we are reminded that dementia is not simply a condition of ageing but can also affect people in mid-life (young onset) also heralds hope since it reflects a shift away from ageist thinking where in the past dementia was seen exclusively as an inevitable aspect of ageing. The life course approach also severs the connections held between dementia and mental health, links that in the past had the potential to reinforce stigma. This is an exciting time for dementia as it means that as a health condition it will no longer sit on the margins but instead, will be incorporated into a much broader debate on issues including primary, secondary and tertiary prevention.

The new approach reminds us that brain health in later life is embedded in physical and mental health in earlier life, so that every stage of the life course is so important (Wu et al, 2016). Policies that target whole populations, such as prevention policies, health promotion and healthcare provision through all stages of life, are also likely to be important (Wu et al, 2016). The public health approach, including the life course framing of dementia, provides opportunities for dementia to share resources with other illness groups (Travers et al, 2015), which means that health promotion strategies applied to other illnesses such as healthy ageing initiatives, chronic disease policies and cardiovascular policies can also now be applied to dementia.

Disability and reablement

At a more micro level and in the absence of an immediate cure for dementia, the disability lens as discussed in Chapter Two of this book also augurs hope. First, the lens shines a strong light on 'excess' or 'unnecessary disabilities', generally more tractable and responsive to interventions than the 'neurological impairment' caused by the disease. Earlier chapters showed how the individual can experience excess disabilities through nihilistic attitudes and through dehumanizing and discriminatory practices, and such attitudes and practices can make life significantly more difficult (Shakespeare et al, 2017), especially if stigma, marginalization, social exclusion and at times, a 'social death', occur. Like a person with a disability, an individual with a cognitive impairment can receive 'oppressive care', support that is over-protective, verging on the paternalistic (Post, 2000). The person can also receive purely technical, task-centred and instrumental care (McLean, 2007) delivered out of a sense of duty, with no attempt made to consider the individual as a relational and emotional human being (Post, 2000).

Oppressive care along with task-centred instrumental care, can contribute to 'excess disability' by ignoring any scope a person has for self-determination, choice, control and autonomy. Much of this type of 'excess disability' could be eliminated if dementia was reframed, nihilistic attitudes eliminated, if the physical environment was more creatively adapted (Marshall, 2001), and if practitioners were better supported through training and mentoring. None of these remedies need to be particularly resource-intensive. Dementia is a significant and growing human problem that needs to be conceptualized as a problem for humanity, and one that entails a collective positive response.

In keeping with the framing of dementia as a disability, the reablement philosophy introduced in earlier chapters (see Chapters Four and Five) also heralds hope for the future since it challenges negative discourse, is well aligned with human rights thinking, focuses positively on what people can still do, with appropriate supports, and empowers the individual 'to gain or restore autonomy in their own space...' (Mishra and Barratt, 2017, p 4). The approach emphasises the importance of early multidisciplinary assessment, and respects and draws on the expertise of a diverse range of health service professionals whose goal is to empower and maximise the individual's functional ability. It takes cognizance of both the person's deficits and strengths, life stories and biographies, and can be used both in community settings and in care homes. The reablement approach means that responsibility for service delivery requires a community focus and must extend beyond the healthcare system. The approach is inclusive of all interventions likely to have a positive impact on the individual's quality of life, including the ethical use of assistive technologies, cognitive rehabilitation and cognitive stimulation therapies. Countries' reimbursement policies must work towards ensuring that the individual and family members have fair and equitable access to both pharmacological and non-pharmacological interventions.

A life of quality and equality

Although the CRPD Articles reviewed in this book relate to human rights, many of these rights as, for example, privacy, independent living, autonomy, choice and participation also constitute important domains of quality of life (Verdugo et al, 2012). Most importantly Article 12, which extends legal capacity to a person with a disability like dementia, cross-cuts all other rights and opens up for the individual new zones of freedom (Quinn, 2010). The Article entitles the person to be treated equally before the law and to have their rights to autonomy respected. The Article means that autonomy can no longer be viewed as a binary concept (full autonomy or no autonomy) that requires rational thinking for its execution. The Article means that a diagnosis of dementia can never be used to restrict a person's autonomy rights nor can it be used to justify the deprivation of a person's legal capacity. Article 12 along with Article 19, which entitles a person to choose their place of residence and have the assistance needed to support living and inclusion in the community, have much potential to promote personhood and to return choice, agency and control, back to the individual provided resources are available (O'Shea and Carney, 2017). The Article has yet to be tested by the person living with dementia, their family members or other representative groups.

Promoting dignity

Respect for the individual's dignity and personhood is a theme that has underpinned much of the material presented in preceding chapters. Dignity is a multifaceted concept and is said to be more easily identified by its absence rather than by its presence (Tadd et al, 2010). It is closely related to notions of autonomy (Nuffield Council on Bioethics, 2009), to privacy (Manthorpe et al, 2010), to quality of life (Kane et al, 2003), to personhood (McLean, 2007) and to upholding the individual's human rights (Nordenfelt, 2004). Respect for dignity is often reflected in how things get done rather than what gets done, and in those little nameless acts, such as a gentle knock on a resident's bedroom door before entrance, dressing the resident in her or his own favourite clothes, the tone of voice used to address that person and most importantly, the humanity with which support is delivered (Nuffield Council on Bioethics, 2009).

Mann (1998) elaborates on dignity violations and refers to the indignity of (i) not being seen, (ii) being seen but only as a group member, (iii) assaults on dignity arising due to personal space being violated and (iv) 'humiliation'. Nordenfelt (2003) identifies four types of dignity, namely (i) 'intrinsic dignity' or *menschenwurde*, which he contends is universal and can never be lost as long as a person is alive; (ii) 'dignity of merit', based on our formal position or ranking in society; (iii) 'dignity of moral stature', based on the individual's moral value; and (iv) 'dignity of identity', which reflects a person's inner experience of dignity. It is the latter component of dignity that he contends is most likely to be affected when a person develops a dementia. As argued earlier in this book, loss of dignity can arise for a whole variety of reasons including, poorly designed care environments, care systems inadequately funded, untrained staff and service limitations (UNECE, 2015b). A just and human society is one that never disempowers, mocks or banishes those who are most vulnerable. It is a society that treats fellow human beings with dignity and respect.

The way forward

Policy

New legislation is insufficient to bring about the social and political change required in dementia services, and much more than the CRPD is needed to ensure that the individual's human rights are respected, promoted and fulfilled. As argued in Chapter Six, policy also needs to be reframed, and governments need to develop plans that reflect a strong commitment to social change and use the new global action plan on dementia (WHO, 2016) to guide policy development. Traditionally policy-makers have framed dementia in negative terms (O'Shea et al, 2015), and the legacy of this type of deficit thinking has permeated government policy. A new human rights approach would sever linkages with this type of deficit thinking (Quinn, 2013a). The key questions would no longer be how can costs be reduced and behaviour controlled, but rather, how can policy be reframed to help a person flourish (Post, 2000), and how can policies be developed that promote strengths, assets, choice, control, autonomy, equality, active participation, personhood (O'Shea et al, 2015) and human rights?

Whilst as noted in Chapter Six the recasting of dementia policy has already started, with some evidence of new frameworks permeating countries' policy plans, the changes apparent reflect recognition of civil and political rights (cost neutral) as opposed to social and economic rights that will be resource-intensive. There is a need for greater commitment on the part of governments to develop policies that promote social and economic rights. At the moment, in most countries, the right to choose where to live is mitigated against by lack of social rights embedded in government policy. Although the new global action plan does not explicitly address the topic of entitlement to social rights, the principle, 'universal health and social care coverage for dementia' (WHO, 2016, p 6), has the potential to be used by dementia activists and the dementia community when campaigning for policy and legislative reform in this area.

Practice

The dementia workforce requires more adequate support (WHO, 2012; Bowers, 2014; OECD, 2015). Practitioners working in dementia care settings are often not well prepared for the multiple challenges supporting a person with more moderate to severe dementia presents. Daily they must deal with complex ethical dilemmas (Alzheimer Europe, 2011) to which there are no easy solutions and for which, in many cases, they have had very limited training (Bowers, 2014). Ethics support (Bollig et al, 2015), a strong management culture (Brooker and Latham, 2016), positive risk-benefit analysis (Nuffield Council on Bioethics, 2009) and ongoing educational programmes that bring the best available evidence-based care to the attention of practitioners (Winblad et al, 2016) and that demonstrate the merits of adopting a biopsychosocial approach to dementia (Revolta et al, 2016) along with applying human rights principles to practice (Kelly and Innes, 2012) are urgently needed.

The need for healthcare professionals and care workers to be more cognizant of human rights was discussed in Chapter Six. That chapter also presented new findings based on practitioners' views of human rights and dementia. It was argued that the PANEL principles underpinning a human rights approach to practice build on elements of person-centred care, and should be used by practitioners to help them interrogate quality of care, question inequities in service provision and reframe and improve practice (Kelly and Innes, 2012). A rights-based framework can also be used by practitioners to request better working conditions and better pay awards. Article 4, which calls for the education of professional staff about human rights, should be used by practitioners to protect their own rights along with user rights, and to hold organizations to account.

Research priorities

Dementia research is said to account for only 0.8 per cent of all public spending on research and development (OECD, 2015). Much of the current research focus is clinical and biomedical, and is concerned with epidemiological, genetic and preventive studies (Alzheimer's Society, 2013a; Batsch, 2016; Winblad et al, 2016) where, if successful, results may benefit future generations but are unlikely to yield much advantage to current generations for whom care and support may be more immediately relevant. Across Europe basic biomedical research when compared with research on care services receives a disproportionately high slice of the dementia research budget (JPND, 2011), even though this type of research takes much time to conduct and results can be disappointing. For example, returns on drug trials remain very low. Cummings et al (2014) showed that in a review of all drug trials registered over a 10-year period, 98 per cent of all phase three trials were unsuccessful. Winblad et al (2016) have also recently cautioned researchers to the risks of launching expensive phase three drug trials without adequate proof of concept.

There is a need for much more transparency on how decisions about research priorities are made (Nuffield Council on Bioethics, 2009); countries need to identify their own research priorities (WHO, 2012) and to learn more from each other about their respective successes and failures. There is also a need for a more balanced research agenda, for more multidisciplinary research and for international collaboration (WHO, 2012; Winblad et al, 2016). Research findings must be made accessible to all, including self-advocates (McDonald and Raymaker, 2013). There is also a need for a greater emphasis to be placed on social science research that has at the fore a clear focus on human rights and ethical frameworks, as this type of research is likely to benefit current generations.

Throughout the chapters of this book I have attempted to highlight areas fruitful for future research, mainly from a social science perspective. These include:

- Longitudinal studies yielding empirical evidence (rather than expert opinion) of the effect of the timing of a dementia diagnosis on the subsequent disease course.
- Cross-sectional studies using large sample sizes investigating how assistive/surveillance technology may advance personhood, promote independence and autonomy and enhance quality of life.
- Evaluation research exploring the potential impact that dementia-friendly communities have on outcome variables including social engagement, active participation, quality of life and time to nursing home admission.
- Cost-benefit analyses of different long-term care models and in particular, studies investigating the financial costs of small-scale households versus more traditional nursing home models of long-term care.
- Research studies examining the unmet needs of individuals with severe dementia in order to identify interventions likely to improve quality of life.

Undoubtedly some of these areas will prove exceptionally challenging to investigate and will pose significant practical, ethical and methodological dilemmas for researchers. Creative designs will be required including in the case of research with people who have mild to moderate dementia, a greater emphasis on narrative techniques (Keady et al, 2007) and on participative action research and discourse analysis. In the context of undertaking research involving the individual with advanced dementia, research instruments will need to be adapted and made available in alternative formats, and more creative thinking applied to devise optimal ways of communicating with the individual (McDonald and Raymaker, 2013).

Conclusion

While the case for risk reduction, prevention and disease-modifying drugs for dementia is undeniable, expectations in the short term for a cure may be unrealistic, given how dementia is not a single disease entity, but rather a syndrome, which at present defies biomedical science, and which describes disparate diseases with different pathophysiology, biochemistry and genetic causes. Hence a magic bullet biomedical solution is unlikely to meet expectations. Therefore the greatest potential benefit to the individual and family members lies in supporting people through relevant economic, health and social policies.

This book has shown how across the world, countries are at different stages in their policy response to dementia. Some, like Scotland, Norway, the US and Australia, have now progressed to second and third iterations of their policy plans. Scotland's third national dementia strategy (2017-2020) (Scottish Government, 2017), which is heavily rights-based, now guarantees a link worker and one-year post-diagnostic services to all persons diagnosed with dementia, a target to which other countries like Australia now aspire (Rees, 2017). Scotland's history of developing its own standards of care for dementia, its own charter of rights and its success in demonstrating how user engagement with policy-makers can make a difference is one that other countries can emulate. The Norwegian *Dementia plan 2020* (Norwegian Government, 2016) places a strong emphasis on human rights, on dignity, self-respect and the right of the individual to choose how to live their own life. The detailed attention the plan pays to the built environment and the importance of small-scale residential units that encourage social interaction and give the individual control over their lives is inspirational. Japan trailblazes the world, having been the first country globally to initiate a dementia friend's programme, now adopted by several other nations. It also leads the world in the development of technology for people living with dementia. In 2013, China ran a most successful media campaign addressing stigma by raising awareness of dementia.

Ireland has been fortunate to have received, in recent years, significant philanthropic funding to support the development and implementation of its first national dementia strategy (DoH, 2014). By providing supports to strengthen capacity and foster leadership qualities in the right people, The Atlantic Philanthropies has shown how quickly the dementia service landscape, previously dominated by a biomedical framing of dementia, can be transformed, with a much stronger emphasis in Ireland today being placed on biopsychosocial models of dementia care (O'Shea and Carney, 2016). Atlantic's investment programme in Ireland has recently been extended to support an ambitious training initiative designed to prevent dementia and produce world leaders in brain health (see, the Global Brain Health Institute at www.gbhi.org). Sweden maintains the largest register of people with dementia in the world (Religa et al, 2015), and the largest register of people with behavioural and psychological symptoms of dementia. Given the respective policy emphasis in different countries, lessons can be learned for those countries new to the development of national strategies and others updating pre-existing strategies.

But no matter how impressive national dementia strategies are, the empirical research reviewed for this book, including first person accounts from the individual and family members, remind us that even in countries brandishing well thought-through policy plans, significant gaps exist between the rhetoric of government policy and the everyday life experiences of the individual living with the symptoms of dementia and their family members who support them. There is strong evidence to suggest that we cannot afford to be complacent. We must seek new and more ethical frameworks to contextualise the debate, develop policy and design services. What is clear is that there is a massive underfunding of all services for people living with dementia. If we believe in human rights, we will not tolerate this current lack of investment in dementia services, and the appeal here is for more realistic resources to be assigned to dementia to enable the individual and family members to exercise their human rights and enjoy a good quality of life.

Finally, it is important to state that in writing this book, the aim has been to open up the debate, ask provocative questions, challenge conventional thinking and raise consciousness about the advantages of conceptualizing dementia as a disability and a rights-based issue. Rather than considering the CRPD as an abstract instrument of no consequence to the lives of persons diagnosed with dementia or their family members, my goal has been to operationalize several of its Articles thereby demonstrating their relevance. I have also attempted to use the CRPD as a prism for enhancing our understanding of dementia and as a tool for social change thereby informing more equitable policy and practice. In her role as former UN Human Rights Commissioner, Mary Robinson, former President of Ireland, once said, "I want to take human rights out of their box. I want to show the relevance of the universal principles of human rights to the basic needs of health, security, education and equality." I hope this book has in some small way achieved this goal for some of the 47 million people around the world today and their family members living with dementia.

References

Adams, T. (1996) 'Kitwood's approach to dementia and dementia care: A critical but appreciative review', *Journal of Advanced Nursing*, vol 23, no 5, pp 948-53.

ADI (2011) *World Alzheimer report 2011: The benefits of early diagnosis and intervention*, London: ADI (www.alz.co.uk/ADI-conference-2011).

ADI (2012) *World Alzheimer report 2012: Overcoming the stigma of dementia*, London: ADI (www.alz.co.uk/research/world-report-2012).

ADI (2013) *World Alzheimer report 2013: An analysis of long-term care for dementia,* London: ADI (www.alz.co.uk/research/world-report-2013).

ADI (2014) *World Alzheimer report 2014: Dementia and risk reduction,* London: ADI (www.alz.co.uk/research/world-report-2014).

ADI (2015a) *World Alzheimer report 2015: The global impact of dementia: An analysis of prevalence, incidence, cost and trends,* London: ADI (www.alz.co.uk/research/world-report-2015).

ADI (2015b) *Dementia-friendly communities* (www.alz.co.uk/dementia-friendly-communities).

African Union (no date) *Protocol to the African Convention on Human and People's Rights on the Rights of Older Persons* (https://au.int/sites/default/files/treaties/31391-sl-protocol_to_the_african_charter_on_human_and_peoples_rights_on_the_rights_of_older_persons.pdf).

AHRC (Australian Human Rights Commission) (2014) *What are human rights?* (www.humanrights.gov.au/about/what-are-human-rights).

Albrecht, G.L., Seelman, K.D. and Bury, M. (eds) (2001) *Handbook of disability studies*, London: Sage Publications.

Allan, K. and Killick, J. (2008) 'Communication and relationships: An inclusive social world', in M. Downs and B. Bowers (eds) *Excellence in dementia care: Research into practice*, Milton Keynes: Open University Press, pp 212–29.

Alston, P. and Megret, F. (2008) *The United Nations and human rights: A critical appraisal*, Oxford: Oxford: University Press.

Altman, B.M. (2001) 'Disability definitions, models, classification schemes, and applications', in G.L. Albrecht, K.D. Seelman and M. Bury (eds) *Handbook of disability studies*, London and New Delhi: Sage Publications, pp 97-122.

Alzheimer Europe (2006) *Paris Declaration on dementia: Public health priorities*, Luxembourg: Alzheimer Europe (www.alzheimer-europe. org/Policy-in-Practice2/Paris-Declaration-2006/Public-health-priorities).

Alzheimer Europe (2010) *Annual report 2010: The ethical issues linked to the use of assistive technology in dementia care*, Luxembourg: Alzheimer Europe.

Alzheimer Europe (2011) *Annual report 2011: The ethics of dementia research*, Luxembourg: Alzheimer Europe.

Alzheimer Europe (2012) *Annual report 2012: The ethical issues linked to restrictions of freedom of people with dementia*, Luxembourg: Alzheimer Europe.

Alzheimer Europe (2013) *National policies covering the care and support of people with dementia and their carers*, Luxembourg: Alzheimer Europe.

Alzheimer Europe (2014a) *Dementia in Europe yearbook: National care pathways for people with dementia living at home*, Luxembourg: Alzheimer Europe.

Alzheimer Europe (2014b) *Glasgow Declaration 2014* (www.alzheimer-europe.org/Policy-in-Practice2/Glasgow-Declaration-2014).

Alzheimer Europe (2015) *Dementia in Europe yearbook: Is Europe becoming more dementia friendly?*, Luxembourg: Alzheimer Europe.

Alzheimer Europe (2016) *Dementia in Europe yearbook: Decision-making and legal capacity issues in dementia*, Luxembourg: Alzheimer Europe.

Alzheimer's Association (2012) '2012 Alzheimer's disease facts and figures', *Alzheimer's & Dementia*, vol 8, no 2, pp 131-68.

Alzheimer's Australia (2014) *Dementia language guidelines* (https:// fightdementia.org.au/files/NATIONAL/documents/language-guidelines-full.pdf).

Alzheimer's Society (2007) *Dementia UK update*, London: Alzheimer's Society (www.alzheimers.org.uk/site/scripts/download_info. php?downloadID=1491).

Alzheimer's Society (2013a) *Cause, cure, care and prevention: Impact of Alzheimer's Society's dementia research programme 1990-2012*, London: Alzheimer's Society.

Alzheimer's Society (2013b) *Low expectations: Attitudes on choice, care and community for people with dementia in care homes*, London: Alzheimer's Society (www.alzheimers.org.uk/site/scripts/download_info. php?fileID=1628).

Alzheimer's Society (2013c) *Building dementia-friendly communities: A priority for everyone*, London: Alzheimer's Society (http://www. actonalz.org/sites/default/files/documents/Dementia_friendly_communities_full_report.pdf)

Amieva, H., Robert, P.H., Grandoulier, A.-S., Meillon, C., de Rotrou, J., Andrieu, S. et al (2016) 'Group and individual cognitive therapies in Alzheimer's disease: The ETNA3 randomized trial', *International Psychogeriatrics*, vol 28, no 5, pp 707-717. doi:10.1017/S1041610215001830 PMID: 26572551

Andrews, J. and Robinson, L. (2013) 'The role of assistive technology in the care of people with dementia', in H. de Waal, C. Lyketsos, D. Ames and J. O'Brien (eds) *Designing and delivering dementia services*, Oxford: John Wiley & Sons, pp 229-239.

Andrews, T. (2012) 'What is social constructionism?', *Grounded Theory Review: An International Journal*, vol 1, no 11.

Annan, K. (2006) 'Statement: Secretary-General's message on the adoption of the Convention of the Rights of Persons with Disabilities', Delivered by Mr Mark Malloch Brown, Deputy Secretary-General, New York: United Nations, 13 December.

Appelbaum, P.S. and Grisso, T. (1995) 'The MacArthur Treatment Competence Study. I: Mental illness and competence to consent to treatment', *Law and Human Behavior*, vol 19, no 2, pp 149-74.

Argyle, E., Downs, M. and Tasker, J. (2010) *Continuing to care for people with dementia: Irish family carers' experience of their relative's transition to a nursing home*, The Alzheimer Society of Ireland, University of Bradford and St Luke's Home (www.alzheimer.ie/Alzheimer/media/SiteMedia/PDF's/Research/Continuing-to-care-for-people-with-dementia.pdf?ext=.pdf).

Arstein-Kerslake, A. and Flynn, E. (2016) 'General Comment on Article 12 of the Convention on the Rights of Persons with Disabilities: A roadmap for equality before the law', *The International Journal of Human Rights*, pp 1-20.

Arthanat, S., Nochajski, S.M. and Stone, J. (2004) 'The international classification of functioning, disability and health and its application to cognitive disorders', *Disability and Rehabilitation*, vol 26, no 4, pp 235-45.

ASI (The Alzheimer Society of Ireland) (2011) 'National dementia summit', unpublished report, Dublin.

ASI (2013) *Human rights and older people in Ireland*, Policy Paper, Dublin (http://alzheimer.ie/Alzheimer/media/SiteMedia/ImageSlider/Fixed/ASI-HROP-A4-Online-Report.pdf).

ASI (2016) *A charter of rights for people with dementia*, Dublin: ASI.

ASPE (Office of the Assistant Secretary for Planning and Evaluation) (2013) *National plan to address Alzheimer's disease: 2013 update*, Washington, DC: ASPE (https://aspe.hhs.gov/national-plan-address-alzheimers-disease-2013-update#strategy3.D).

ASPE (2016) *National plan to address Alzheimer's disease: 2016 update*, Washington, DC: ASPE (https://aspe.hhs.gov/report/national-plan-address-alzheimers-disease-2016-update).

Assisted Decision-Making (Capacity) Act (Ireland) (2015) (www.irishstatutebook.ie/eli/2015/act/64/enacted/en/html)

Astell, A. (2006) 'Technology and personhood in dementia care', *Quality in Ageing and Older Adults*, vol 7, no 1, pp 15-25.

Audit Commission (2003) *Human rights: Improving public service delivery*, London: Audit Commission.

Ausserhofer, D., Deschodt, M., De Geest, S., van Achterberg, T., Meyer, G., Verbeek, H. et al (2016) '"There's no place like home": A scoping review on the impact of homelike residential care models on resident-, family-, and staff-related outcomes', *Journal of the American Medical Directors Association*, vol 17, no 8, pp 685-93.

Australian Government Department of Health (2015) *National framework for action on dementia 2015-2019*, Ageing and Aged Care (https://agedcare.health.gov.au/ageing-and-aged-care-older-people-their-families-and-carers-dementia/national-framework-for-action-on-dementia-2015-2019).

Bail, K.D. (2003) 'Electronic tagging of people with dementia: Devices may be preferable to locked doors', *BMJ*, vol 326, no 7383, p 281.

Baker, C. (2015) *Developing excellent care for people living with dementia in care homes*, London: Jessica Kingsley Publishers.

Baldwin, C. and Capstick, A. (2007) *Tom Kitwood on dementia: A reader and critical commentary*, London: McGraw-Hill Education.

Ballard, C., Hanney, M.L., Theodoulou, M., Douglas, S., McShane, R., Kossakowski, K. et al (2009) 'The dementia antipsychotic withdrawal trial (DART-AD): Long-term follow-up of a randomised placebo-controlled trial', *The Lancet Neurology*, vol 8, no 2, pp 151-7.

Bamford, C., Lamont, S., Eccles, M., Robinson, L., May, C. and Bond, J. (2004) 'Disclosing a diagnosis of dementia: A systematic review', *International Journal of Geriatric Psychiatry*, vol 19, no 2, pp 151-69.

Banerjee, S. (2009) *The use of antipsychotic medication for people with dementia: Time for action*, A report for the Minister of State for Care Services, London: Department of Health (www.rcpsych.ac.uk/pdf/Antipsychotic%20Bannerjee%20Report.pdf).

Banerjee, S. (2010) 'Living well with dementia: Development of the National Dementia Strategy for England', *International Journal of Geriatric Psychiatry*, vol 25, pp 917-22.

Banerjee, S. (2013) 'Developing policy that works for dementia: National and global lessons in what makes a difference', in H. de Waal, C. Lyketsos, D. Ames and J. O'Brien (eds) *Designing and delivering dementia services*, Oxford: Wiley Blackwell, pp 119-25.

Banerjee, S. (2015) 'A narrative review of evidence for the provision of memory services', *International Psychogeriatrics*, vol 27, no 10, pp 1583-92.

Barnes, C. (1991) *Disabled people in Britain and discrimination: A case for anti-discrimination legislation*, London: C. Hurst & Co. Publishers.

Barnes, C. and Mercer, G. (2010) *Exploring disability* (2nd edn), Bodmin: MPG Books Group.

Bartlett, R. (2000) 'Dementia as a disability: Can we learn from disability studies and theory?', *Journal of Dementia Care*, Sept/Oct, pp 33-36.

Bartlett, R. (2014) 'Citizenship in action: The lived experiences of citizens with dementia who campaign for social change', *Disability & Society*, vol 29, no 8, pp 1291-304.

Bartlett, R. (2016) 'Scanning the conceptual horizons of citizenship', *Dementia*, vol 15, no 3, pp 453-61.

Bartlett, R. and O'Connor, D. (2007) 'From personhood to citizenship: Broadening the lens for dementia practice and research', *Journal of Ageing Studies*, vol 21, pp 107-18.

Bartlett, R. and O'Connor, D. (2010) *Broadening the dementia debate: Towards social citizenship*, Bristol: Policy Press.

Batsch, N. (2016) 'Conceptualizing empowerment from the perspectives of people with mild dementia', Unpublished PhD thesis, King's College London.

Beard, R.L. (2012) 'Art therapies and dementia care: a systematic review', *Dementia*, vol 11, no 5, pp 633-56.

Beattie, A.M., Daker-White, G., Gilliard, J. and Means, R. (2005) 'They don't quite fit the way we organise our services' – Results from a UK field study of marginalised groups and dementia care', *Disability & Society*, vol 20, no 1, pp 67-80.

Begley, E. (2009) 'I know what it is but how bad does it get? Insights into the lived experience and service needs of people with early-stage dementia', PhD, Trinity College, Dublin, Ireland.

Benoit, M., Arbus, C., Blanchard, F., Camus, V., Cerase, V., Clement, J.P. et al (2006) 'Professional consensus on the treatment of agitation, aggressive behaviour, oppositional behaviour and psychotic disturbances in dementia', *The Journal of Nutrition, Health & Aging*, vol 10, no 5, pp 410-15.

Bewley, C. (1998) *Tagging: A technology for care services?*, London: Values into Action.

BIHR (British Institute of Human Rights) (2010) *Your human rights: A guide for older people*, London: BIHR.

Bjørneby, S., Topo, P., Cahill, S., Begley, E., Jones, K., Hagen, I. et al (2004) 'Ethical considerations in the ENABLE project', *Dementia: The International Journal of Social Research and Practice*, vol 3, no 3, pp 297-312.

Black, B.S. and Rabins, P.V. (2013) 'Services for people with severe dementia', in H. de Waal, C. Lyketsos, D. Ames and J. O'Brien (eds) *Designing and delivering dementia services*, Oxford: John Wiley & Sons, pp 90-102.

Black, B.S., Johnston, D., Morrison, A., Rabins, P.V., Lyketsos, C.G. and Samus, Q.M. (2012) 'Quality of life of community-residing persons with dementia based on self-rated and caregiver-rated measures', *Quality of Life Research*, vol 21, no 8, pp 1379-89.

Blackman, T., Mitchell, L., Burton, E., Jenks, M., Parsons, M., Raman, S. and Williams, K. (2003) 'The accessibility of public spaces for people with dementia: A new priority for the "open city"', *Disability & Society*, vol 18, no 3, pp 357-71.

Blessed G., Tomlinson, B.E. and Roth, M. (1968) 'The association between quantitative measures of dementia and of senile change in the cerebral grey matter of elderly subjects', *The British Journal of Psychiatry*, vol 114, no 512, pp 797-811.

Bobersky, A. (2013) 'It's been a good move. Transitions into care: Family caregivers', persons with dementia, and formal staff members' experiences of specialist care unit placement', Unpublished PhD thesis, Trinity College, Dublin, Ireland.

Boekhorst, S.T., Depla, M.F.I.A., Francke, A.L., Twisk, J.W.R., Zwijsen, S.A. and Hertogh, C.M.P.M. (2013) 'Quality of life of nursing home residents with dementia subject to surveillance technology versus physical restraints: an explorative study', *International Journal of Geriatric Psychiatry*, vol 28, no 4, pp 356-63.

Boïse, L., Morgan, D.L., Kaye, J. and Camicioli, R. (1999) 'Delays in the diagnosis of dementia: Perspectives of family caregivers', *American Journal of Alzheimer's Disease and Other Dementias*, vol 14, no 1, pp 20-6.

Bollig, G., Schmidt, G., Rosland, J.H. and Heller, A. (2015) 'Ethical challenges in nursing homes – Staff's opinions and experiences with systematic ethics meetings with participation of residents' relatives', *Scandinavian Journal of Caring Sciences*, vol 29, no 4, pp 810-23.

Bond, J. (1992) 'The medicalization of dementia', *Journal of Aging Studies*, vol 6, no 4, pp 397-403.

Bond, J. (2001) 'Sociological perspectives', in C. Cantley (ed) *A handbook of dementia care*, Buckingham: Open University Press, pp 44-61.

Bond, J., Corner, L., Lilley, A. and Ellwood, C. (2002) 'Medicalization of insight and caregivers' responses to risk in dementia', *Dementia: The International Journal of Social Research and Practice*, vol 1, pp 313-28.

Boustani, M., Perkins, A.J., Fox, C., Unverzagt, F., Austrom, M.G., Fultz, B. et al (2006) 'Who refuses the diagnostic assessment for dementia in primary care?', *International Journal of Geriatric Psychiatry*, vol 21, no 6, pp 556-63.

Bowers, (2014) A trained and supported workforce, in M. Downs and B. Bowers (eds) *Excellence in dementia care – research into practice*, second edition, Open University Press, Berkshire, England, pp 417-29.

Boyle, G. (2008) 'Autonomy in long-term care: A need, a right or a luxury', *Disability & Society*, vol 23, no 4, pp 299-310.

Boyle, G. (2010) 'Social policy for people with dementia in England: Promoting human rights?', *Health & Social Care in the Community*, vol 18, no 5, pp 511-19.

Bradshaw, J. (1972) 'A taxonomy of social need', in G. McLachlan (ed) *Problems and progress in medical care: essays on current research* (7th series), Oxford: University Press, London, pp 71-82.

Bradshaw, J. (1994) 'The conceptualisation and measurement of need: A social policy perspective', in J. Popay and G. Williams (eds) *Researching the people's health*, London: Routledge, pp 45-57.

Bradshaw, S., Playford, D. and Riazi, A. (2012) 'Living well in care homes: A systematic review of qualitative studies', *Age and Ageing*, vol 41, no 4, pp 429-40.

Brannelly, T. (2011) 'Sustaining citizenship: People with dementia and the phenomenon of social death', *Nursing Ethics*, vol 18, no 5, pp 662-71.

Brawley, E. (2001) 'Environmental design for Alzheimer's disease: A quality of life issue', *Aging & Mental Health*, vol 5, S1, pp 79-83.

Brisenden, S. (1986) 'Independent living and the medical model of disability', *Disability & Society*, vol 1, no 2, pp 173-8.

Brock, D.W. (1988) 'Justice and the severely demented elderly', *Journal of Medicine and Philosophy*, vol 13, no 1, pp 73-99.

Brodaty, H. and Cumming, A. (2010) 'Dementia services in Australia', *International Journal of Geriatric Psychiatry*, vol 25, no 9, pp 887-995.

Brooker, D.J. (2001) 'Therapeutic activity', in C. Cantley (ed) *A handbook of dementia care*, Buckingham: Open University Press, pp 146-59.

Brooker, D.J. (2004) 'What is person centred care for people with dementia?', *Reviews in Clinical Gerontology*, vol 13, no 3, pp 215-22.

Brooker, D.J. and Latham, I. (2016) *Person-centred dementia care: Making services better with the VIPS framework*, London: Jessica Kingsley Publishers.

Brooker, D.J., Fontaine, J.L., Evans, S., Bray, J. and Saad, K. (2014) 'Public health guidance to facilitate timely diagnosis of dementia: Alzheimer's Cooperative Valuation in Europe recommendations', *International Journal of Geriatric Psychiatry*, vol 29, no 7, pp 682-93.

Brooker, D.J., Latham, I., Evans, S.C., Jacobson, N., Perry, W., Bray, J. et al (2016) 'FITS into practice: Translating research into practice in reducing the use of anti-psychotic medication for people with dementia living in care homes', *Aging & Mental Health*, vol 20, no 7, pp 709-18.

Browning, M., Bigby, C. and Douglas, J. (2014) 'Supported decision making: Understanding how its conceptual link to legal capacity is influencing the development of practice', *Research and Practice in Intellectual and Developmental Disabilities*, vol 1, no 1, pp 34-45.

Bryden, C. (2015) *Nothing about us without us: 20 years of dementia advocacy*, London and Philadelphia, PA: Jessica Kingsley Publishers.

Bulmer, M. (2015) *The social basis of community care (Routledge Revivals)*, London: Routledge.

Burns, A.S., Guthrie, E., Marino-Francis, F., Busby, C., Morris, J., Russell, E. et al (2005) 'Brief psychotherapy in Alzheimer's disease: Randomised controlled trial', *British Journal of Psychiatry*, vol 187, pp 143-7.

Bökberg, C., Ahlström, G., Leino-Kilpi, H., Soto-Martin, M.E., Cabrera, E., Verbeek, H. et al (2015) 'Care and service at home for persons with dementia in Europe', *Journal of Nursing Scholarship*, vol 47, no 5, pp 407-16.

Cadigan, R.O., Grabowski, D.C., Givens, J.L. and Mitchell, S.L. (2012) 'The quality of advanced dementia care in the nursing home: The role of special care units', *Medical Care*, vol 50, no 10, p 856.

Cahill, S. (1997) '"I wish I could have hung on longer": Choices and dilemmas in dementia care', PhD thesis, University of Queensland, Australia.

Cahill, S. (2010) 'Developing a national dementia strategy for Ireland', *International Journal of Geriatric Psychiatry*, vol 9, pp 912-16.

Cahill, S. and Diaz-Ponce, A. (2011) '"I hate having nobody here, I'd like to know where they all are": Can qualitative research detect differences in quality of life among nursing home residents with different levels of cognitive impairment?', *Ageing and Mental Health*, vol 15, no 5, pp 562-72.

Cahill, S. and Diaz-Ponce, A. (2017) Quality of life of members of a religious community living in long term care', *Perspectives on science and Christian faith*, vol 69, no 4, pp 206-16.

Cahill, S. and Dooley, A. (2005) 'The historical context of rehabilitation and its application to dementia care', in M. Marshall (ed) *Perspectives on rehabilitation and dementia*, London and Philadelphia, PA: Jessica Kingsley Publishers, pp 30-8.

Cahill, S. and Pierce, M. (2013) *Briefing paper on dementia diagnosis*, Genio, Ireland.

Cahill, S. and Rosenman, L. (1991) 'Caregiver considerations in institutionalising dementia patients', in D. O'Neill (ed) *Carers, professionals and Alzheimer's disease,* London: Libbey & Co, pp 37-42.

Cahill, S., Begley, E., Topo, P., Saarikalle, K., Macijauskiene, J., Budraitiene, A. et al (2004) '"I know where this is going and I know it won't go back": Hearing the individual's voice in dementia quality of life assessments', *Dementia*, vol 3, no 3, pp 313-30.

Cahill, S., Clark, M., Walsh, C., O'Connell, H. and Lawlor, B. (2006) 'Dementia in primary care: The first survey of Irish general practitioners', *International Journal of Geriatric Psychiatry*, vol 21, no 4, pp 319-24.

Cahill, S., Clark, M., O' Connell, H., Lawlor, B., Coen, R.F. and Walsh, C. (2008) 'The attitudes and practices of general practitioners regarding dementia diagnosis in Ireland', *International Journal of Geriatric Psychiatry*, vol 23, no 7, pp 663-69.

Cahill, S., Diaz-Ponce, A.M., Coen, R.F. and Walsh, C. (2010) 'The under-detection of cognitive impairment in nursing homes in the Dublin area. The need for ongoing cognitive assessment', *Age and Ageing*, vol 39, no 1, pp 128-31.

Cahill, S., O'Shea, E. and Pierce, M. (2012) *Creating excellence in dementia care: A research review for Ireland's National Dementia Strategy*, DSIDC's Living with Dementia Research Programme, Dublin and Galway: School of Social Work and Social Policy, Trinity College, Dublin and Irish Centre for Social Gerontology, National University of Ireland.

Cahill, S., Pierce, M. and Bobersky, A. (2014a) *An evaluation report on the dementia support worker initiative of the 5 steps to living well with dementia in South Tipperary Project*, Genio, Ireland.

Cahill, S., Pierce, M. and Moore, V. (2014b) 'A national survey of memory clinics in the Republic of Ireland', *International Psychogeriatrics*, vol 26, no 4, pp 605-13.

Cahill, S., O'Nolan, C., O'Caheny, D. and Bobersky, A. (2015a) *An Irish national survey of dementia in long term residential care*, Dublin: Dementia Services Information and Development Centre (www.dementia.ie/images/uploads/site-images/DSIDCReport_439721.pdf).

Cahill, S., Pierce, M., Werner, P., Darley, A. and Bobersky, A. (2015b) 'A systematic review of the public's knowledge and understanding of Alzheimer's disease and dementia', *Alzheimer Disease & Associated Disorders*, vol 29, no 3, pp 255-75.

Calkins, M.P. (1988) *Design for dementia: Planning environments for the elderly and the confused*, Owings Mills, MD: National Health Publishing.

Calkins, M.P., Szmerekovsky, J.G. and Biddle, S. (2007) 'Effect of increased time spent outdoors on individuals with dementia residing in nursing homes', *Journal of Housing for the Elderly*, vol 21, no 3-4, pp 211-28.

Cantley, C. (2001) *A handbook of dementia care*, Buckingham: Open University Press.

Cantley, C. and Bowes, A. (2004) 'Dementia and social inclusion: The way forward', in A. Innes, C. Archibald and C. Murphy (eds) *Dementia and social inclusion: Marginalized groups and marginalized areas of dementia research, care and practice*, London: Jessica Kingsley Publishers, pp 255-71.

Cantley, C. and Smith, G. (2001) 'Research, policy and practice in dementia care', in C. Cantley (ed) *A handbook of dementia care*, Buckingham: Open University Press, pp 295-308.

Capezuti, E. (2004) 'Minimizing the use of restrictive devices in dementia patients at risk for falling', *Nursing Clinics of North America*, vol 39, no 3, pp 625-47.

Carboni, J.T. (1990) 'Homelessness among the institutionalized elderly', *Journal of Gerontological Nursing*, vol 16, no 7, pp 32-7.

Cash, M. (2003) 'Assistive technology and people with dementia', *Reviews in Clinical Gerontology*, vol 13, no 4, pp 313-19.

Castle, N.G. (2006) 'Mental health outcomes and physical restraint use in nursing homes', *Administration and Policy in Mental Health and Mental Health Services Research*, vol 33, no 6, p 696.

Cayton, H. (2006) *Report of the Ministerial Taskforce on the NHS Summary Care Record*, London: Connecting for Health (www. connectingforhealth.nhs.uk/resources/care_record_taskforce_doc. pdf).

Chan, M. (2015) *Final statement of the Director General of WHO: First WHO ministerial conference on global action against dementia*, Geneva, Switzerland: United Nations Human Rights, Office of the High Commissioner for Human Rights.

Chung, J.C.C. and Lai, C.K.Y. (2002) 'Snoezelen for dementia', e Cochrane Database of Systematic Reviews, DOI: 10.1002/14651858. CD003152.

Charlton, J.I. (1998) *Nothing about us without us: Disability oppression and empowerment*, Berkeley, CA: University of California Press.

Charlton, J.I. (2000) *Nothing about us without us: Disability oppression and empowerment*, London: University of California Press.

Cheek, P., Nikpour, L. and Nowlin, H.D. (2005) 'Aging well with smart technology', *Nursing Administration Quarterly*, vol 29, no 4, pp 329-38.

Clapham, A. (2007) *Human rights: A very short introduction*, Oxford: Oxford University Press.

Clare, L. (2003) 'Managing threats to self: awareness in early stage Alzheimer's disease', *Social Science & Medicine*, vol 57, pp 1017-29.

Clare, L. (2017) 'Rehabilitation for people living with dementia: A practical framework of positive support', *PLOS Medicine*, vol 14, no 3.

Clare, L. and Woods, R.T. (2004) 'Cognitive training and cognitive rehabilitation for people with early-stage Alzheimer's disease: A review', *Neuropsychological Rehabilitation*, vol 14, pp 385-401.

Clare, L., Marková, I., Verhey, F. and Kenny, G. (2005) 'Awareness in dementia: A review of assessment methods and measures', *Aging & Mental Health*, vol 9, no 5, pp 394-413.

Clare, L., Quinn, C., Hoare, Z., Whitaker, R. and Woods, R.T. (2014) 'Care staff and family member perspectives on quality of life in people with very severe dementia in long-term care: A cross-sectional study', *Health and Quality of Life Outcomes*, vol 12, no 1, p 175.

Clare, L., Bayer, A., Burns, A., Corbett, A., Jones, R., Knapp, M. et al (2013) 'Goal-oriented cognitive rehabilitation in early-stage dementia: Study protocol for a multi-centre single-blind randomised controlled trial (GREAT)', *Trials*, vol 14, no 1, p 152.

Clarke, C.L., Keyes, S.E., Wilkinson, H., Alexjuk, J., Wilcockson, J., Robinson, L. et al (2013) *Healthbridge, the national evaluation of peer support networks and dementia advisers in the implementation of the National Dementia Strategy for England*, London: Department of Health Policy Research Programme Project.

Coen, R., Flynn, B., Rigney, E., O'Connor, E., Fitzgerald, L., Murray, C. et al (2011) 'Efficacy of a cognitive stimulation therapy programme for people with dementia', *Irish Journal of Psychological Medicine*, vol 28, no 3, pp 145-7.

Cohen, D. and Eisdorfer, C. (1986) *The loss of self: A family resource for the care of Alzheimer's disease disorders*, New York and London: W.W. Norton & Company.

Cohen, U. and Weisman, G.D. (1991) *Holding on to home: Designing environments for people with dementia*, Baltimore, MD: Johns Hopkins University Press.

Cohen-Mansfield, J., Marx, M.S., Thein, K. and Dakheel-Ali, M. (2011) 'The impact of stimuli on affect in persons with dementia', *The Journal of Clinical Psychiatry*, vol 72, no 4, p 480.

Connell, C.M., Boise, L., Stuckey, J.C., Holmes, S.B. and Hudson, M.L. (2004) 'Attitudes toward the diagnosis and disclosure of dementia among family caregivers and primary care physicians', *The Gerontologist*, vol 44, no 4, pp 500-7.

Convery, J. (2014) 'Here today gone tomorrow: An exploratory study of housing with care development for people with dementia in Ireland', Unpublished PhD thesis, Trinity College, Dublin, Ireland.

Cook, A.M. and Polgar, J.M. (2014) *Assistive technologies: Principles and practice*, St. Louis, MO: Elsevier Health Sciences.

Coon, J.T., Abbott, R., Rogers, M., Whear, R., Pearson, S., Lang, I. et al (2014) 'Interventions to reduce inappropriate prescribing of antipsychotic medications in people with dementia resident in care homes: A systematic review', *Journal of the American Medical Directors Association*, vol 15, no 10, pp 706-18.

Cooper, C., Mukadam, N., Katona, C., Lyketsos, G.C., Ames, D., Rabins, P. et al (2012) 'Systematic review of the effectiveness of non-pharmacological interventions to improve quality of life of people with dementia', *International Psychogeriatrics*, vol 24, pp 856-70.

Corner, L. and Bond, J. (2004) 'Being at risk of dementia: Fears and anxieties of older adults', *Journal of Aging Studies*, vol 18, no 2, pp 143-55.

CORU (2011) *Code of professional conduct and ethics for social workers*, Social Workers Registration Board, Dublin, Ireland.

Council of Europe, Steering Committee for Human Rights (CCDH), *Recommendation CM/Rec (2014)2 of the Committee of Ministers to Member States on the promotion of the human rights of older persons CM/ Rec (2014)2* (www.coe.int/t/dghl/standardsetting/hrpolicy/other_ committees/cddh-age/Document_CDDH_AGE/CMRec(2014)2_ en.pdf).

Crespo, M., de Quirós, M.B., Gómez, M.M. and Hornillos, C. (2012) 'Quality of life of nursing home residents with dementia: A comparison of perspectives of residents, family, and staff', *The Gerontologist*, vol 52, no 1, pp 56-65.

Crowther, N. (2015) 'Dementia, human rights and the social model of disability', Making Rights Make Sense blog, 28 September (https:// makingrightsmakesense.wordpress.com).

Cummings, J.L., Morstorf, T. and Zhong, K. (2014) 'Alzheimer's disease drug-development pipeline: Few candidates, frequent failures', *Alzheimer's Research & Therapy*, vol 6, no 4, p 37.

DAI (Dementia Alliance International) (2016) *The human rights of people living with dementia: From rhetoric to reality*, Ankeny, IA: DAI (www. alzheimers.org.nz/getattachment/News-Info/Global-information/ Human-Rights-for-People-Living-with-Dementia-Rhetoric-to- Reality.pdf).

Dautzenberg, P.L., van Marum, R.J., van der Hammen, R. and Paling, H.A. (2003) 'Patients and families desire a patient to be told the diagnosis of dementia: A survey by questionnaire on a Dutch memory clinic', *International Journal of Geriatric Psychiatry*, vol 18, no 9, pp 777-9.

Deal, M. (2003) 'Disabled people's attitudes toward other impairment groups: A hierarchy of impairments', *Disability & Society*, vol 18, no 7, pp 897-910.

Degener, T. (2014) 'A human rights model of disability', *Disability Social Rights* (www.researchgate.net/publication/283713863_A_ human_rights_model_of_disability).

de Lange, J., Willemse, B., Smit, D. and Pot, A.M. (2011) 'Housing with care for people with dementia in the Netherlands', a paper delivered at seminar at Trinity College, Dublin, Nov 2011.

de Lepeleire, J., Wind, A.W., Iliffe, S., Moniz-Cook, E.D., Wilcock, J., González, W.M. et al (2008) 'The primary care diagnosis of dementia in Europe: An analysis using multidisciplinary, multinational expert groups', *Aging & Mental Health*, vol 12, no 5, pp 568-76.

Dementia Forum X (2015) '*An international initiative focusing on the global challenges of dementia*' (http://dementiaforumx.org/).

Demenz (2013) *Demenz: Rapport final du Comité de pilotage en vue de l'établissement d'un plan d'action national – maladies démentielles*, Le Gouvernement du Grand-Duché de Luxemburg (www.mfi.public. lu/a_z/D/Demence/RapportFinal.pdf).

Denzin, N.K. and Lincoln, Y.S. (1994) *Handbook of qualitative research*, Michigan, MI: Sage Publications, University of Michigan.

de Siún, A., O'Shea, E., Timmons, S., McArdle, D., Gibbons, P., O'Neill, D. et al (2014) *Irish national audit of dementia care in acute hospitals*, Dublin: University College Cork and Trinity College, Dublin (www.ucc.ie/en/media/research/irishnationalauditofdementia/ INADFullReportLR.pdf).

Dewing, J. (2008) 'Personhood and dementia: Revisiting Tom Kitwood's ideas', *International Journal of Older People Nursing*, vol 3, no 1, pp 3-13.

DH (Department of Health, UK) (2009) *Living well with dementia: A national dementia strategy*, London: DH (www.gov.uk/government/ publications/living-well-with-dementia-a-national-dementia-strategy).

DH (2015) *Prime Minister's challenge on dementia 2020*, London: DH (www.gov.uk/government/uploads/system/uploads/attachment_ data/file/414344/pm-dementia2020.pdf).

Dhanda, A. (2006) 'Legal capacity in the disability rights convention: Stranglehold of the past or lodestar for the future', *Syracuse Journal of International Law and Commerce*, vol 34, p 429.

Dhedhi, S.A., Swinglehurst, D. and Russell, J. (2014) '"Timely" diagnosis of dementia: What does it mean? A narrative analysis of GPs' accounts', *BMJ Open*, vol 4, no 3, e004439.

DHSSPS (Department of Health Social Services and Public Safety) (2011) *Improving dementia services in Northern Ireland: A regional strategy* (www.health-ni.gov.uk/sites/default/files/publications/dhssps/ improving-dementia-services-2011.pdf).

DHSSPS (Department of Health Social Services and Public Safety) (2015) *Care standards for nursing homes*, Belfast: DHSSPS. (www.rqia. org.uk/RQIA/media/RQIA/Resources/Standards/nursing_homes_ standards_-_april_2015.pdf).

Diaz-Ponce, A. (2008) 'Quality of life of people with cognitive impairment living in a residential setting. The subjective views of residents, relatives and staff', Unpublished MSc in Applied Social Research, Trinity College, Dublin, Ireland.

Diaz-Ponce, A. (2014) 'Quality of life and anti-dementia medication: An exploration of the experiences of people living with dementia and their care-partners', Unpublished PhD thesis, Trinity College, Dublin, Ireland.

Diaz-Ponce, A. and Cahill, S. (2013) 'Dementia and quality-of-life issues in older people', in C. Phellas (ed) *Aging in European societies*, New York: Springer, pp 97-115.

Disability Rights UK (2010) *A guide to the UN disability convention*, London: Disability Rights UK (www.disabilityrightsuk.org/policy-campaigns/campaigns/equally-ours-campaign/guide-un-disability-convention).

DoH (2014) *The Irish national dementia strategy*, Dublin: The Stationery Office (http://health.gov.ie/wp-content/uploads/2014/12/30115-National-Dementia-Strategy-Eng.pdf).

Donnelly, J. (2007) 'The relative universality of human rights', *Human Rights Quarterly*, vol 29, no 2, pp 281-306.

Donnelly, S. (2012) 'Family meeting or care planning meeting? A multidisciplinary team action research study in a hospital setting', Unpublished PhD thesis, Trinity College, Dublin, Ireland.

Donnelly, S., O'Brien, M., Begley, E. and Brennan, J. (2016) *'I'd prefer to stay at home but I don't have a choice': Meeting older people's preference for care: Policy, but what about practice?*, Dublin: University College Dublin.

Dorenlot, P. (2005) 'Applying the social model of disability to dementia: Present-day challenges', *Dementia: The International Journal of Social Research and Practice*, vol 4, no 4, pp 459-61.

Downs, M., Small, N. and Froggatt, K. (2006) 'Explanatory models of dementia: Links to end-of-life care', *International Journal of Palliative Nursing*, vol 12, no 5, pp 209-13.

Doyle, P. and Rubinstein, R. (2014) 'Person-centered dementia care and the cultural matrix of othering', *Gerontologist*, vol 54, no 6, pp 952-63.

Dröes, R.M., Boelens-Van der Knoop, E.C., Bos, J., Meihuizen, L., Ettema, T.P., Gerritsen, D.L. Hoogeveen, F., De Lange, J. and Schölzel-Dorenbos, C.J.M. (2006) 'Quality of life in dementia in perspective An explorative study of variations in opinions among people with dementia and their professional caregivers, and in literature', *Dementia*, vol 5, no 4, pp 533-58.

Dupuis, S.L., Kontos, P., Mitchell, G. and Gray, J. (2016) 'Re-claiming citizenship through the arts', *Dementia*, vol 15, no 3, pp 358-80.

Edvardsson, D., Sandman, P.O., Nay, R. and Karlsson, S. (2009) 'Predictors of job strain in residential dementia care nursing staff', *Journal of Nursing Management*, vol 17, no 1, pp 59-65.

EHRC (2010) 'The United Nations Convention on the rights of people with disabilities. What does it mean for you?: A guide for disabled people and disabled people's organisations', Equality and Human Rights Commission (EHRC), Manchester, England. https://www.equalityhumanrights.com/sites/default/files/the-united-nations-convention-on-the-rights-of-persons-with-disabilities-what-does-it-mean-for-you.pdf

Eley, M. (2016) 'Telling it as it is: Involving people with dementia and family carers in policy making, service design and workforce development', *Working with Older People*, vol 20, no 4, pp 219-22.

EMA (European Medicines Agency) (2008) *Questions and answers on the review of the use of conventional antipsychotic medicines in elderly patients with dementia* (www.ema.europa.eu/docs/en_GB/document_library/Other/2010/01/WC500054058.pdf).

Engedal, K. (2005) 'Assessment of dementia and use of anti-dementia drugs in nursing homes', *Tidsskrift for den Norske Laegeforening: Tidsskrift for Praktisk Medicin, Ny Raekke*, vol 125, no 9, pp 1188-90.

ENNHRI (European Network of National Human Rights Institutions) (2016) *The CRPD and older people with disabilities: The transition to community-based long-term care services* (www.ennhri.org/IMG/pdf/policy_brief_final_version-2.pdf).

EPWD (European Parliament Written Declaration) (2009) *Call for joint EU action on Alzheimer's and Parkinson's* (http://www.europarl.europa.eu/sides/getDoc.do?type=IM-PRESS&reference=20091110IPR64183&format=XML&language=EN)

Estes, C.L., Biggs, S. and Phillipson, C. (2003) *Social theory, social policy and ageing*, Maidenhead: Open University Press.

Ettema, T.P., Dröes, R.M., de Lange, J., Ooms, M.E., Mellenbergh, G.J. and Ribbe, M.W. (2005) 'The concept of quality of life in dementia in the different stages of the disease', *International Psychogeriatrics*, vol 17, no 3, pp 353-70.

EU (European Union) FRA (Agency for Fundamental Rights) (2013a) *Fundamental rights: Challenges and achievements in 2013 – Annual report 2013* (http://fra.europa.eu/en/publication/2014/fundamental-rights-challenges-and-achievements-2013-annual-report-2013).

EU FRA (2013b) *Legal capacity of persons with intellectual disabilities and persons with mental health problem* (http://fra.europa.eu/en/publication/2013/legal-capacity-persons-intellectual-disabilities-and-persons-mental-health-problems).

Eurobarometer (2007) Special 283, *Health and long-term care in the EU*, European Commission.

European Parliament (2011) *European initiative on Alzheimer's disease* (www.europarl.europa.eu/sides/getDoc.do?type=TA&language=EN&reference=P7-TA-2011-0016).

Fang, R., Ye, S., Huangfu, J. and Calimag, D.P. (2017) 'Music therapy is a potential intervention for cognition of Alzheimer's disease: A mini-review', *Translational Neurodegeneration*, vol 6, no 1, p 2.

Federal Office of Public Health (Switzerland) (2016) *Swiss national dementia strategy 2014-2019* (www.bag.admin.ch/bag/en/home/themen/strategien-politik/nationale-gesundheitsstrategien/nationale-demenzstrategie-2014-2017.html).

Fetherstonhaugh, D., Tarzia, L. and Nay, R. (2013) 'Being central to decision making means I am still here! The essence of decision making for people with dementia', *Journal of Aging Studies*, vol 27, no 2, pp 143-50.

Finnema, E., Droes, R.M., Ribbe, M. and van Tilburg, W. (2000) 'A review of psychosocial models in psychogeriatrics: Implications for care and research', *Alzheimer Disease and Associated Disorders*, vol 14, pp 68-80.

Fisk, J.D., Beattie, B.L., Donnelly, M., Byszewski, A. and Molnar, F.J. (2007) 'Sure of the diagnosis of dementia', *Alzheimer's & Dementia*, vol 3, no 4, pp 404-10.

Fleissig, A., Jenkins, V., Catt, S. and Fallowfield, L. (2006) 'Multidisciplinary teams in cancer care: Are they effective in the UK?', *The Lancet Oncology*, vol 7, no 11, pp 935-43.

Fleming, R. and Sum, S. (2014) 'Empirical studies on the effectiveness of assistive technology in the care of people with dementia: A systematic review', *Journal of Assistive Technologies*, vol 8, no 1, pp 14-34.

Flynn, E. (2011) *From rhetoric to action: Implementing the UN Convention on the Rights of Persons with Disabilities*, Cambridge: Cambridge University Press.

Flynn, E. and Arstein-Kerslake, A. (2014) 'Legislating personhood: Realising the right to support in exercising legal capacity', *International Journal of Law in Context*, vol 10, no 1, pp 81-104.

Foebel, A.D., Onder, G., Finne-Soveri, H., Lukas, A., Denkinger, M.D., Carfi, A. et al (2016) 'Physical restraint and antipsychotic medication use among nursing home residents with dementia', *Journal of the American Medical Directors Association*, vol 17, no 2, pp 184-e9-14.

Foley, T.D., Swanwick, G.P. (2014) *Dementia-diagnosis and management in general practice: Quick reference guide*, Lenus: The Irish Health Repository.

Forbat, L. (2006) 'An analysis of key principles in Valuing People: Implications for supporting people with dementia', *Journal of Intellectual Disabilities*, vol 10, no 3, pp 249-60.

Forrester, L.T., Maayan, N., Orrell, M., Spector, A.E., Buchan, L.D. and Soares-Weiser, K. (2014) 'Aromatherapy for dementia', *The Cochrane Library*.

Forsythe, D.P. (2012) *Human rights in international relations*, Cambridge: Cambridge University Press.

Fortinsky, R. and Downs, M. (2014) 'Optimizing person-centred transitions in the dementia journey: A comparison of national dementia strategies', *Health Affairs*, vol 33, no 4, pp 566-73.

Fossey, J., Ballard, C., Juszczak, E., James, I., Alder, N., Jacoby, R. and Howard, R. (2006) 'Effect of enhanced psychosocial care on antipsychotic use in nursing home residents with severe dementia: Cluster randomized trial', *British Medical Journal*, vol 332, pp 756-61.

French Plan Maladies Neuro-Degeneratives (2014-2019) *Plan Maladies Neuro-Degeneratives*, Strategie Nationale de Sante', France (www.alzheimer-europe.org/Policy-in-Practice2/National-Dementia-Strategies/France)

G8 Summit (2013) Official documents (www.g8.utoronto.ca/summit/2013lougherne/).

Gabel, M.J., Foster, N.L., Heidebrink, J.L., Higdon, R., Aizenstein, H.J., Arnold, S.E. et al (2010) 'Validation of consensus panel diagnosis in dementia', *Archives of Neurology*, vol 67, no 12, pp 1506-12.

García Iriarte, E. (2016) 'Models of disability', in E. García Iriarte, R. McConkey and G. Gilligan (eds) *Disability and human rights*, New York: Palgrave Macmillan, pp 10-30.

García Iriarte, E., McConkey, R. and Gilligan R. (2016) *Disability and human rights*, New York: Palgrave Macmillan.

Gardner, H. and Barraclough, S. (1992) *The policy process. Health policy development, implementation and evaluation in Australia*, Melbourne, VIC: Churchill Livingstone.

Gauri, V. and Gloppen, S. (2012) 'Human rights-based approaches to development: Concepts, evidence, and policy', *Polity*, vol 44, no 4, pp 485-503.

George, D.R. (2010) 'Overcoming the social death of dementia through language', *The Lancet*, vol 76, no 9741, pp 586-7.

Georges, J. (2013) 'Making dementia a European priority', in H. de Waal, C. Lyketsos, D. Ames and J. O'Brien (eds) *Designing and delivering dementia services*, Oxford: John Wiley & Sons, pp 111-14.

Georges, J., Jansen, S., Jackson, J., Meyrieux, A., Sadowska, A. and Selmes, M. (2008) 'Alzheimer's disease in real life – The dementia carer's survey', *International Journal of Geriatric Psychiatry*, vol 23, no 5, pp 546-51.

Gergen, K.J. (2009) *Realities and relationships: Soundings in social construction*, Cambridge, MA: Harvard University Press.

Gibson, F. (2011) *Reminiscence and life story work: A practice guide*, London: Jessica Kingsley Publishers.

Gibson, G., Dickinson, C., Brittain, K. and Robinson, L. (2015) 'The everyday use of assistive technology by people with dementia and their family carers: A qualitative study', *BMC Geriatrics*, vol 15, no 1.

Gilliard, J. and Marshall, M. (2012) *Transforming the quality of life for people with dementia through contact with the natural world: Fresh air on my face*, London and Philadelphia, PA: Jessica Kingsley Publishers.

Gilliard, J., Means, R., Beattie, A. and Daker-White, G. (2005) 'Dementia care in England and the social model for disability – Lessons and issues', *Dementia: The International Journal of Social Research and Practice*, vol 4, no 4, pp 571-86.

Gilmour, J.A. and Brannelly, T. (2010) 'Representations of people with dementia – Subaltern, person, citizen', *Nursing Inquiry*, vol 17, no 3, pp 240-7.

Gilson, S.F. and Depoy, E. (2000) 'Multiculturalism and disability: A critical perspective', *Disability & Society*, vol 15, no 2, pp 207-18.

Girardet, T.H. and Schumacher, S. (1999) *Creating sustainable cities*, Totnes: Green Books, for the Schumacher Society.

Gjerberg, E., Hem, H.M., Førde, R. and Pedersen, R. (2013) 'How to avoid and prevent coercion in nursing homes: A qualitative study', *Nursing Ethics*, vol 20, no 6, pp 632-44.

Goffman, E. (1963) *Behavior in public places*, Glencoe, IL: Free Press.

Goodley, D. (2001) '"Learning difficulties", the social model of disability and impairment: Challenging epistemologies', *Disability & Society*, vol 16, no 2, pp 207-31.

Goodley, D. (2011) *Disability studies: An interdisciplinary introduction*, London: Sage.

Goodley, D. and Runswick-Cole, K. (2011) 'The violence of disablism', *Sociology of Health & Illness*, vol 33, no 4, pp 602-17.

Gove, D., Downs, M., Vernooij-Dassen, M. and Small, N. (2015) 'Stigma and GPs' perceptions of dementia', *Aging & Mental Health*, vol 20, no 4, pp 1-10.

Grand, J., Casper, S. and MacDonald, S. (2011) 'Clinical features and multidisciplinary approaches to dementia care', *Journal of Multidisciplinary Healthcare*, vol 4, pp 125-47.

Gray-Vickrey, P. (2009) 'Media coverage of persons with Alzheimer's disease', *Alzheimer's Care Today*, vol 10, no 2, pp 57-8.

Grossetete, F. Bowis J., Lévai, K. Tadeusz Masiel, J. and Trakatellis, A. (2008) 0080/2008 European Parliament Written Declaration on priorities in the fight against Alzheimer's disease.

Gubrium, J.F. (1986) *Oldtimers and Alzheimer's*, Greenwich, CT: JAI Press: Greenwich, Connecticut.

Guleria, R. and Curtice, M. (2015) 'Dementia, rights and the social model of disability' (www.rcpsych.ac.uk/workinpsychiatry/ faculties/oldagepsychiatry/newsletters/enewsletterjanuary2016/ dementiaandrights.aspx).

Hagen, I., Holthe, T., Gilliard, J., Topo, P., Cahill, S., Begley, E. et al (2004) 'Development of a protocol for the assessment of assistive aids for people with dementia', *Dementia*, vol 3, no 3, pp 281-96.

Hamers, J.P. and Huizing, A.R. (2005) 'Why do we use physical restraints in the elderly?', *Zeitschrift für Gerontologie und Geriatrie*, vol 38, no 1, pp 19-25.

Hamers, J.P., Gulpers, M.J. and Strik, W. (2004) 'Use of physical restraints with cognitively impaired nursing home residents', *Journal of Advanced Nursing*, vol 45, no 3, pp 246-51.

Hammersley, M. (2014) 'The perils of impact for academic social science', *Contemporary Social Science*, vol 9, no 3, pp 345-55.

Happell, B. (2005) 'Mental health nursing: Challenging stigma and discrimination towards people experiencing a mental illness', *International Journal of Mental Health Nursing*, vol 14, no 1, pp 1-1.

Harding, R. and Peel, E. (2013) '"He was like a zombie": Off-label prescription of antipsychotic drugs in dementia', *Medical Law Review*, vol 21, no 2, pp 243-77.

Hare, P. (2016) *Our dementia, our rights*, Exeter: Dementia Engagement and Empowerment Project (DEEP) and Innovations in Dementia CIC.

Harmer, B.J. and Orrell, M. (2008) 'What is meaningful activity for people with dementia living in care homes? A comparison of the views of older people with dementia, staff and family carers', *Aging & Mental health*, vol 12, no 5, pp 548-58.

Harris-Kojetin, L., Sengupta, M., Park-Lee, E. and Valverde, R. (2013) 'Long-term care services in the United States: 2013 overview', *Vital & Health Statistics. Series 3, Analytical and Epidemiological Studies*/US Department of Health and Human Services, Public Health Service, National Center for Health Statistics, vol 37, pp 1-107.

Hazzan, A.A., Humphrey, J., Kilgour-Walsh, L., Moros, K.L., Murray, C., Stanners, S. et al (2016) 'Impact of the "artful moments" intervention on persons with dementia and their care partners: A pilot study', *Canadian Geriatrics Journal*, vol 19, no 2, p 1.

Heggestad, A.K.T., Nortvedt, P. and Slettebø, Å. (2013) '"Like a prison without bars": Dementia and experiences of dignity', *Nursing Ethics*, vol 20, no 8, pp 881-92.

HelpAge International (2015) *A new Convention on the Rights of Older People: A concrete proposal* (http://social.un.org/ageing-working-group/documents/sixth/HelpAgeInternational.pdf).

HM Government of Gibraltar (2015) *National dementia vision and strategy for Gibraltar* (www.gibraltar.gov.gi/new/sites/default/files/HMGoG_Documents/HMGoG%20National%20Dementia%20Vision%20and%20Strategy.pdf).

Hofmann B. (2013) 'Ethical challenges with welfare technology: A review of the literature', *Science and Engineering Ethics*, vol 19, no 2, pp 389-406.

Holicky, R. (1996) 'Caring for the caregivers: The hidden victims of illness and disability', *Rehabilitation Nursing*, vol 21, no 5, pp 247-52.

House of Commons (2007) *The human rights of older people in healthcare*, House of Lords, House of Commons, Joint Committee on Human Rights, London: The Stationery Office Limited (publications.parliament.uk/pa/jt200607/jtselect/jtrights/156/156i.pdf).

Howorth, P. and Saper, J. (2003) 'The dimensions of insight in people with dementia', *Aging & Mental Health*, vol 7, no 2, pp 113-22.

HSE (Health Service Executive) (2016) Dementia Understand Together campaign (www.hse.ie/eng/services/list/4/olderpeople/dementia/About-Understand-Together/nationaldementiaoffice/nationaldementiastrategy/).

Hughes, J. (2011) *Thinking through dementia: International perspectives in philosophy and psychiatry*, Oxford: Oxford University Press.

Hughes, J. (2014) *How we think about dementia: Personhood, rights, ethics, the arts and what they mean for care*, London: Jessica Kingsley Publishers.

Hughes, J. and Louw, S (2002) 'Electronic tagging of people with dementia who wander: Ethical considerations are possibly more important than practical benefits', *BMJ*, vol 325, no 7369, pp 847-8.

Hughes, R. (2010) 'Human rights perspectives', in R. Hughes (ed) *Rights, risks and restraint-free care of older people: Person-centred approaches in health and social care*, London: Jessica Kingsley Publishers, pp 97-104.

Hulko, W. and Stern, L. (2009) 'Cultural Safety, Decision-Making and Dementia: Troubling notions of autonomy and personhood', in D. O'Connor and B. Purves (eds) *Decision-making, personhood and dementia: Exploring the interface*, Jessica Kingsley Publishers, London, pp 70-87.

Hunter, C. and Doyle, C. (2014) 'Dementia policy in Australia and the social construction of infirm old age', *Australian and New Zealand Society of the History of Medicine*, vol 16, no 2, pp 44-62.

Hyman, M.A. (2008) 'Does dementia exist? Dispelling the myth', *Alternative Therapies in Health and Medicine*, vol 14, no 2, p 10.

Ife, J. (2012) *Human rights and social work: Towards rights-based practice*, New York: Cambridge University Press.

Iliffe, S. and Manthorpe, J. (2004) 'The debate on ethnicity and dementia: From category fallacy to person-centred care?', *Aging & Mental Health*, vol 8, no 4, pp 283-92.

Iliffe, S. and Wilcock, J. (2005) 'The identification of barriers to the recognition of, and response to, dementia in primary care using a modified focus group approach', *Dementia*, vol 4, no 1, pp 73-85.

Iliffe, S., de Lepeleire, J., van Hout, H., Kenny, G., Lewis, A., Vernooij-Dassen, M.J.F.J. and The Diadem Group (2005) 'Understanding obstacles to the recognition of and response to dementia in different European countries: A modified focus group approach using multinational, multi-disciplinary expert groups', *Aging & Mental Health*, vol 9, no 1, pp 1-6.

Iliffe, S., Robinson, L., Brayne, C., Goodman, C., Rait, G., Manthorpe, J. and Ashley, P. (2009) 'Primary care and dementia: 1. Diagnosis, screening and disclosure', *International Journal of Geriatric Psychiatry*, vol 24, no 9, pp 895-901.

Ilinca, S., Leichsenring, K. and Rodrigues, R. (2015) 'From care in homes to care at home: European experiences with (de) institutionalisation in long-term care', Policy brief, European Centre.

IMH (2013) *Addressing Alzheimer's and other types of dementia: Israeli national strategy*, Jerusalem: Ministry of Health (www.health.gov.il/PublicationsFiles/Dementia_strategy-Eng.pdf).

Imogen Blood and Associates (2017) *Evidence review of dementia-friendly communities*, European Union Joint Action on Dementia.

Innes, A. (2009) *Dementia studies*, London: Sage Publications.

Innes, A. and Manthorpe, J. (2013) 'Developing theoretical understandings of dementia and their application to dementia care policy in the UK', *Dementia*, vol 12, no 6, pp 682-96.

Innes, A., Archibald, C. and Murphy, C. (2004) *Dementia and social inclusion: Marginalised groups and marginalised areas of dementia research, care and practice*, London: Jessica Kingsley Publishers.

Innes, A., McCabe, L. and Watchman, K. (2012) 'Caring for older people with an intellectual disability: A systematic review', *Maturitas*, vol 72, no 4, pp 286-95.

INS (2013) *National Programme for Addressing Alzheimer's and other types of dementia*, Israeli national strategy, Ministry of Health.

Irish Human Rights and Equality Commission Act (2014) (www. irishstatutebook.ie/eli/2014/act/25/enacted/en/html).

Irish Examiner (2015) 'Special report: Dementia in Ireland – We must tackle risks at earlier age', 25 June.

Irish Times (2015) 'Dementia rate falls as health-conscious men "become more like women"', 20 April (www.irishtimes.com/news/health/dementia-rate-falls-as-health-conscious-men-become-more-like-women-1.2617275).

Janus, S.I., van Manen, J.G., IJzerman, M.J. and Zuidema, S.U. (2016) 'Psychotropic drug prescriptions in Western European nursing homes', *International Psychogeriatrics*, pp 1-16.

Jarrott, S.E., Kwack, H.R. and Relf, D. (2002) 'An observational assessment of a dementia-specific horticultural therapy program', *HortTechnology*, vol 12, no 3, pp 403-10.

Jennings, B. (2010) 'Agency and moral relationship in dementia', in E.F. Kittay and L. Carlson (eds), *Cognitive disability and its challenge to moral philosophy*, Chichester: Wiley-Blackwell Publishers, pp 171-82.

Jing, W., Willis, R. and Feng, Z. (2016) 'Factors influencing quality of life of elderly people with dementia and care implications: A systematic review', *Archives of Gerontology and Geriatrics*, vol 66, pp 23-41.

Jones, A. and May, J. (1996) *Working in human service organizations: A critical introduction*, Melbourne, VIC: Longman.

Jones, P. (2000) 'Individuals, communities and human rights', *Review of International Studies*, vol 26, no 5, pp 199-215.

Jones, R.W. (2013) 'Services for people with mild dementia', in H. de Waal, C. Lyketsos, D. Ames and J. O'Brien (eds) *Designing and delivering dementia services*, Oxford: Wiley & Sons Ltd, pp 60-72.

Jönson, H. and Larsson, A.T. (2009) 'The exclusion of older people in disability activism and policies – A case of inadvertent ageism?', *Journal of Aging Studies*, vol 23, no 1, pp 69-77.

JPND (2011) *JPND Mapping exercise report*, JPND Research (www. neurodegenerationresearch.eu/initiatives/mapping-excercise/2011-report/).

JPND (2017) 'What research does JPND support?' (www.neurodegenerationresearch.eu/).

Kales, H.C., Gitlin, L.N. and Lyketsos, C.G. (2015) 'State of the art review: Assessment and management of behavioral and psychological symptoms of dementia', *BMJ*, vol 350.

Kane, R.A. (2001) 'Long-term care and a good quality of life: Bringing them closer together', *The Gerontologist*, vol 41, no 3, pp 293-304.

Kane, R.A., Kling, K.C., Bershadsky, B., Kane, R.L., Giles, K., Degenholtz, H.B. et al (2003) 'Quality of life measures for nursing home residents', *The Journals of Gerontology: Series A*, vol 58, no 3, pp M240-8.

Keady, J., Ashcroft-Simpson, S., Halligan, K. and Williams, S. (2007) 'Admiral nursing and the family care of a parent with dementia: Using autobiographical narrative as grounding for negotiated clinical practice and decision-making', *Scandinavian Journal of Caring Sciences*, vol 21, no 3, pp 345-53.

Kelly, F. (2010) 'Abusive interactions: Research in locked wards for people with dementia', *Social Policy and Society*, vol 9, no 2, pp 267-77.

Kelly, F. and Innes, A. (2012) 'Human rights, citizenship and dementia care nursing', *International Journal of Older People Nursing*, vol 8, pp 61-70.

Kelly, M. (2005) *The right not to be ill-treated: A practical guide to the European Convention on Human Rights*, Belfast: Human Rights Commission.

Kelly, M. and O'Sullivan, M. (2015) *Strategies and techniques for cognitive rehabilitation: Manual for healthcare professionals working with people with cognitive impairment*, The Alzheimer Society of Ireland.

Kennerley, D. and de Waal, H. (2013) 'Workforce planning and development', in H. de Waal, C. Lyketsos, D. Ames and J. O'Brien (eds) *Designing and delivering dementia services*, Oxford: Wiley-Blackwell, pp 215-28.

Kidd, J. (2012) 'Commentary on "Human rights training: Impact on attitudes and knowledge"', *Tizard Learning Disability Review*, vol 17, no 2, pp 88-91.

Kim, S. (2015) 'Cognitive rehabilitation for elderly people with early-stage Alzheimer's disease', *Journal of Physical Therapy Science*, vol 27, pp 543-6.

Kinderman, P. and Butler, F. (2006) *Implementing a human rights approach within public services: An outline psychological perspective*, London: Department for Constitutional Affairs.

King's Fund Centre (1986) *Living well into old age: Applying principles of good practice to services for people with dementia*, Report No 63, London: King's Fund Publishing Office.

Kirkevold, Ø. and Engedal, K. (2004) 'Prevalence of patients subjected to constraint in Norwegian nursing homes', *Scandinavian Journal of Caring Sciences*, vol 18, no 3, pp 281-6.

Kitwood, T. (1988) 'The technical, the personal, and the framing of dementia', *Social Behaviour*, vol 3, pp 161-80.

Kitwood, T. (1990) 'The dialectics of dementia: With particular reference to Alzheimer's disease', *Ageing & Society*, vol 10, no 2, pp 177-96.

Kitwood, T. (1993a) 'Person and process in dementia', *International Journal of Geriatric Psychiatry*, vol 8, pp 541-55.

Kitwood, T. (1993b) 'Towards a theory of dementia care: The interpersonal process', *Ageing & Society*, vol 13, no 1, pp 51-67.

Kitwood, T. (1995) 'Positive long-term changes in dementia: Some preliminary observations', *Journal of Mental Health*, vol 4, no 2, pp 133-44.

Kitwood, T. (1997a) *Dementia reconsidered: The person comes first*, Buckingham: Open University Press.

Kitwood, T. (1997b) 'The experience of dementia', *Aging & Mental Health*, vol 1, no 1, pp 13-22.

Kitwood, T. and Bredin, K. (1992) 'Towards a theory of dementia care: Personhood and well-being', *Ageing & Society*, vol 12, pp 269-87.

Knapp, M., Comas-Herrera, A., Somani, A. and Banerjee, S. (2007) *Dementia: International comparisons*, London: LSE/PSSRU, Institute of Psychiatry at the Maudsley, London School of Economics and Political Science.

Koch, T. and Iliffe, S. (2010) 'Rapid appraisal of barriers to the diagnosis and management of patients with dementia in primary care: A systematic review', *BMC Family Practice*, vol 11, no 1, p 1.

Konetzka, R.T., Brauner, D.J., Shega, J. and Werner, R.M. (2014) 'The effects of public reporting on physical restraints and antipsychotic use in nursing home residents with severe cognitive impairment', *Journal of the American Geriatrics Society*, vol 62, no 3, pp 454-61.

Kontos, P.C. and Naglie, G. (2007) 'Bridging theory and practice: Imagination, the body, and person-centred dementia care', *Dementia*, vol 6, no 4, pp 549-69.

Kornfeld-Matte, R. (2015) 'Dementia, a public health priority and a human rights concern', 16 March, Statement to the Ministerial Conference on Global Action against Dementia, Geneva: World Health Organization (unpublished speech).

Landau, R., Auslander, G.K., Werner, S., Shoval, N. and Heinik, J. (2010) 'Families' and professional caregivers' views of using advanced technology to track people with dementia', *Qualitative Health Research*, vol 20, no 3, pp 409-19.

Law Society of Scotland (2013) *Submission to the CRPD Committee on the Draft General Comment on Article 12 CRPD*, November (www.ohchr.org/Documents/HRBodies/CRPD/GC/LawSocietyOfScotlandArt12.doc).

Lawton, M.P. (1977) 'The impact of the environment on aging and behavior', in J.E. Birren and K. Warner Schaie (eds) *Handbook of the Psychology of Aging*, San Diego, CA: Academic Press, pp 276-301.

Lawton, M.P. (2001) 'The physical environment of the person with Alzheimer's disease', *Aging & Mental Health*, vol 5, suppl 1, pp 56-64.

Lawton, M.P., Kleban, M., Moss, M., Rovine, M. and Glicksman, A. (1989) 'Measuring caregiver appraisal', *Journal of Gerontology*, vol 44, no 3, pp 61-71.

Laybourne, A.H., Jepson, M.J., Williamson, T., Robotham, D., Cyhlarova, E. and Williams, V. (2016) 'Beginning to explore the experience of managing a direct payment for someone with dementia: The perspectives of suitable people and adult social care practitioners', *Dementia*, vol 15, no 1, pp 125-40.

Lewis, L. (2009) 'Politics of recognition: What can a human rights perspective contribute to understanding users' experiences of involvement in mental health services?', *Social Policy and Society*, vol 8, no 2, pp 257-74.

Lindemann, H. (2014) 'Second nature and tragedy of Alzheimer's', in L.-C. Hydén, H. Lindemann and J. Brookmeier (eds) *Beyond loss: Dementia, identity, personhood*, Oxford: Oxford Scholarship Online, Oxford University Press, pp 11-23.

Lindenmuth, G.F. and Moose, B. (1990) 'Improving cognitive abilities of elderly Alzheimer's patients with intense exercise therapy', *American Journal of Alzheimer's Care and Related Disorders & Research*, vol 5, no 1, pp 31-3.

Low, L.F., White, F., Jeon, Y.H., Gresham, M. and Brodaty, H. (2013) 'Desired characteristics and outcomes of community care services for persons with dementia: What is important according to clients, service providers and policy?', *Australasian Journal on Ageing*, vol 32, no 2, pp 91-6.

Lyman, K.A. (1989) 'Bringing the social back in: A critique of the biomedicalization of dementia', *The Gerontologist*, vol 29, no 5, pp 597-605.

Magai, C., Cohen, C.I. and Gomberg, D. (2002) 'Impact of training dementia caregivers in sensitivity to nonverbal emotion signals', *International Psychogeriatrics*, vol 14, no 1, pp 25-38.

Malta (2015) *Empowering change, A national strategy for dementia in the Maltese Islands, 2015-2023*, Parliamentary Secretary for the rights of persons with disability and active ageing (www.ceafa.es/files/2017/05/MALTA.pdf).

Mandela, N. (1990) Speech to the joint meeting of Congress, Washington, 26 June.

Mann, J. (1998) 'Dignity and health: The UDHR's revolutionary first article', *Health and Human Rights*, vol 3, no 2, pp 30-38.

Manthorpe, J. and Adams, T. (2003) 'Policy and practice in dementia care', in T. Adams and Manthorpe (eds) *Dementia Care*, pp 35-50.

Manthorpe, J., Illife, S. and Eden, A. (2003) 'Early recognition of dementia by nurses', *Journal of Advanced Nursing*, vol 44, no 2, pp 183-91.

Manthorpe, J., Iliffe, S., Samsi, K., Cole, L., Goodman, C., Drennan, V. and Warner, J. (2010) 'Dementia, dignity and quality of life: Nursing practice and its dilemmas', *International Journal of Older People Nursing*, vol 5, no 3, pp 235-44.

Marks, S.P. (2014) *Human rights: A brief introduction*, Boston, MA: Harvard School of Public Health.

Marshall, M. (1994) 'Emerging trends in dementia care: Some thoughts on the next ten years', Concluding presentation at ADI (Alzheimer's Disease International) conference, Edinburgh, 23 September.

Marshall, M. (1998) 'Therapeutic buildings for people with dementia', in S. Judd, S.P. Phippen, and M. Marshall (eds) *Design for dementia*, *Journal of Dementia Care*, London, pp 11-14.

Marshall, M. (1999) 'What do service planners and policy-makers need from research?', *International Journal of Geriatric Psychiatry*, vol 14, no 2, pp 86-96.

Marshall, M. (2001) 'Care settings and care environments', in C. Cantley (ed) *A handbook of dementia care*, Buckingham: Open University Press, pp 173-86.

Marshall, M. (2003) 'Not just because we do it', *Journal of Dementia Care*, vol 11, no 6, p 10.

Marshall, M. (2005) 'Perspectives on rehabilitation and dementia', in M. Marshall (ed) *Perspectives on rehabilitation and dementia*, London: Jessica Kingsley Publishers, pp 13-19.

Maslow, A. (1970) *Motivation and personality* (2nd edn), New York: Harper Press.

Mattke, S., Klautzer, L. and Mengistu, T. (2011) *Health and well-being in the home: A global analysis of needs, expectations, and priorities for home health care technology*, Rand Corporation.

Maunder, L. (2013) 'Human rights: Equality for all residents in residential nursing homes', *Australian Nursing Journal*, vol 13, no 20, p 8.

McCabe, L. and Bradley, B.E. (2012) 'Supporting user participation in local policy development: The Fife dementia strategy', *Social Policy and Society*, vol 11, no 2, p 157.

McDonald, K.E. and Raymaker, D.M. (2013) 'Paradigm shifts in disability and health: Toward more ethical public health research', *American Journal of Public Health*, vol 103, no 12, pp 2165-73.

McGettrick, G. (2014) 'The UN Disability Convention as an instrument for people with dementia and their carers', Alzheimer Europe Conference, Glasgow.

McGilton, K.S., Davis, A.M., Naglie, G., Mahomed, N., Flannery, J., Jaglal, S. et al (2013) 'Evaluation of patient centred rehabilitation model targeting older persons with a hip fracture including those with cognitive impairment', *BMC Geriatrics*, vol 13, p 136.

McLean, A. (2007) *The person in dementia: A study of nursing home care in the US*, Toronto, BC: University of Toronto Press.

McLean, A. (2010) 'New approaches to nursing home/dementia care in the US: A contextual review', Paper presented at Living with Dementia Seminar, Long Room Hub, Trinity College, Dublin, Ireland, 29 September.

McShane, R., Hope, T. and Wilkinson, J. (1994) 'Tracking patients who wander: Ethics and technology', *The Lancet*, vol 343, no 8908, p 1274.

McSherry, B. (2012) 'Legal capacity under the Convention on the Rights of Persons with Disabilities', *Journal of Law and Medicine*, vol 20, pp 22-7.

Meenan, H., Rees, N. and Doron, I. (2016) 'Introduction', in H. Meenan, N. Rees, and I. Doron (eds) *Towards human rights in residential care for older persons: International perspectives*, London: Routledge, pp 1-12.

Mental Capacity Act (England and Wales) 2005 (www.legislation.gov.uk/ukpga/2005/9/contents).

Mental Health Foundation (2015) *Dementia rights and the social model of disability: A new direction for policy and practice*, London: Mental Health Foundation.

Mills, C.W. (1959) *The sociological imagination*, New York: Oxford University Press.

Milne, A. (2010) 'The 'D' word: Reflections on the relationship between stigma, discrimination and dementia', *Journal of Mental Health*, vol 19, no 3, pp 227-33.

Ministry of Health (France) (2008) *French national plan for 'Alzheimer and related diseases' (2008-2012)*, Paris (www.cnsa.fr/documentation/plan_alzheimer_2008-2012-2.pdf).

Milte, R., Shulver, W., Killington, C., Bradley, C., Ratcliffe, J. and Crotty, M. (2016) 'Quality in residential care from the perspective of people living with dementia: The importance of personhood', *Archives of Gerontology and Geriatrics*, vol 63, pp 9-17.

Mishra, V. and Barratt, J. (2016) 'Reablement and older people', IFA Copenhagen Summit, April 17-19, 2016.

Mitchell, G.J. and Templeton, M. (2014) 'Ethical considerations of doll therapy for people with dementia', *Nursing Ethics*, vol 21, no 6, pp 720-30.

Mitchell, G.J., Dupuis, S.L. and Kontos, P. (2013) 'Dementia discourse: From imposed suffering to knowing other-wise', *Journal of Applied Hermeneutics*, vol 2, article 5, pp 1-19.

Mittelman, M.S., Ferris, S.H., Shulman, E., Steinberg, G. and Levin, B. (1996) 'A family intervention to delay nursing home placement of patients with Alzheimer disease: A randomized controlled trial', *JAMA*, vol 276, no 21, pp 1725-31.

Mittler, P. (2012) 'What can we learn from disability movement', in N. Batsch, M. Mittelman and Alzheimer's Disease International, *World Alzheimer report 2012: Overcoming the stigma of dementia*, London: Alzheimer's Disease International, pp 68-69.

Mittler, P. (2015) 'Time for action: Asserting our rights', *Journal of Dementia Care*, vol 23, no 6, p 10.

Mittler, P. (2016a) 'The UN Convention on the Rights of Persons with Disabilities: Implementing a paradigm shift', in E. García Iriarte, R. McConkey and R. Gilligan (eds) *Disability and human rights*, Basingstoke: Palgrave Macmillan Education, pp 33-48.

Mittler, P. (2016b) 'The United Nations Convention on the Rights of Persons with Disabilities: What does it have to offer people with dementia?', Paper presented at Health Policy Plenary, Annual Conference, Alzheimer's Disease International, Budapest, 23 April.

Mjørud, M., Engedal, K., Røsvik, J. and Kirkevold, M. (2017) 'Living with dementia in a nursing home, as described by persons with dementia: A phenomenological hermeneutic study', *BMC Health Services Research*, vol 17, no 1, p 93.

Moïse, P., Schwarzinger, M. and Um, M. (2004) *Dementia care in 9 OECD countries: A comparative analysis*, OECD Health Working Papers, no 13, Paris: OECD Publishing (http://dx.doi.org/10.1787/485700737071).

Moore, V. and Cahill, S. (2013) 'Diagnosis and disclosure of dementia – A comparative qualitative study of Irish and Swedish general practitioners', *Aging & Mental Health*, vol 17, no 1, pp 77-84.

Morgan, S. and Andrews, N. (2016) 'Positive risk-taking: From rhetoric to reality', *The Journal of Mental Health Training, Education and Practice*, vol 11, no 2, pp 122-32.

Morrissey, F. (2015) 'Assisted Decision-Making Bill: Why changes are needed to current laws', *Irish Examiner*, 21 November.

Moyle, W., Fetherstonhaugh, D., Greben, M. and Beattie, E. (2015) 'Influencers on quality of life as reported by people living with dementia in long-term care: A descriptive exploratory approach', *BMC Geriatrics*, vol 15, no 1, p 50.

Moyle, W., Murfield, J., Venturto, L., Griffiths, S., Grimbeek, P., McAllister, M. and Marshall, J. (2014) 'Dementia and its influence on quality of life and what it means to be valued: Family members' perceptions', *Dementia*, vol 13, no 3, pp 412-25.

Moyle, W., Venturto, L., Griffiths, S., Grimbeek, P., McAllister, M., Oxlade, D. and Murfield, J. (2011) 'Factors influencing quality of life for people with dementia: A qualitative perspective', *Aging & Mental Health*, vol 15, no 8, pp 970-7.

Muñiz, R., Gómez, S., Curto, D., Hernández, R., Marco, B., Garcia, P. et al (2016) 'Reducing physical restraints in nursing homes: A report from María Wolff and Sanitas', *Journal of the American Medical Directors Association*, vol 17, no 7, pp 633-9.

Muò, R., Schindler, A., Vernero, I., Schindler, O., Ferrario, E. and Brisoni, G. (2005) 'Alzheimer's disease-associated disability: An ICF approach', *Disability and Rehabilitation*, vol 27, no 23, pp 1405-13.

Murphy, K. and Welford, C. (2012) 'Agenda for the future: Enhancing autonomy for older people in residential care', *International Journal of Older People Nursing*, vol 7, no 1, pp 75-80.

Murphy, K., O'Shea, E., Cooney, A., Shiel, A. and Hodgins, M. (2006) *Improving quality of life for older people in long-stay care settings in Ireland*, Dublin: National Council on Ageing and Older People.

Nakanishi, M. and Nakashima, T. (2014) 'Features of the Japanese national dementia strategy in comparison with international dementia policies: How should a national dementia policy interact with the public health-and social-care systems?', *Alzheimer's & Dementia*, vol 10, no 4, pp 468-76.

Nedlund, A.C. and Nordh, J. (2015) 'Crafting citizen (ship) for people with dementia: How policy narratives at national level in Sweden informed the politics of the time from 1975 to 2013', *Journal of Aging Studies*, vol 34, pp 123-33.

NICE (National Institute for Health and Clinical Excellence)/SCIE (Social Care Institute for Excellence) (2007) *Dementia: A NICE-SCIE guideline on supporting people with dementia and their carers in health and social care*, National Clinical Practice Guideline No 42, The British Psychological Society and Gaskell, London: NICE/SCIE.

Niemeijer, A.R., Depla, M.F., Frederiks, B.J. and Hertogh, C.M. (2015) 'The experiences of people with dementia and intellectual disabilities with surveillance technologies in residential care', *Nursing Ethics*, vol 22, no 3, pp 307-20.

Niemeijer, A.R., Frederiks, B.J., Riphagen, I.I., Legemaate, J., Eefsting, J.A. and Hertogh, C.M. (2010) 'Ethical and practical concerns of surveillance technologies in residential care for people with dementia or intellectual disabilities: An overview of the literature', *International Psychogeriatrics*, vol 22, no 7, pp 1129-42.

Nilsson, A. (2012) *Who gets to decide? Right to legal capacity for persons with intellectual and psychosocial disabilities*, Issue Paper published by the Council of Europe Commissioner for Human Rights (https://rm.coe.int/16806da5c0).

Nordenfelt, L. (2004) 'The varieties of dignity', *Health Care Analysis*, vol 12, no 2, pp 69-81, discussion 83-9.

Northern Ireland Human Rights Commission (2012) *In defence of dignity: The human rights of older people in nursing homes*, Belfast: Northern Ireland Human Rights Commission (www.nihrc.org/documents/research-and-investigations/older-people/in-defence-of-dignity-investigation-report-March-2012.pdf).

Norwegian Government (2016) *Dementia plan 2020* (www.regjeringen.no/no/dokumenter/demensplan-2020/id2465117/).

Norwegian Ministry of Health and Care Services (2015) *Subplan of care plan 2015: Dementia plan 2015*, Oslo: Government of Norway.

Nuffield Council on Bioethics (2009) *Dementia: Ethical issues*, London: Nuffield Council on Bioethics.

Nursing Home Support Scheme Act (2009) (www.irishstatutebook.ie/eli/2009/act/15/enacted/en/index.html).

Nåden, D., Rehnsfeldt, A., Råholm, M.B., Lindwall, L., Caspari, S., Aasgaard, T. et al (2013) 'Aspects of indignity in nursing home residences as experienced by family caregivers', *Nursing Ethics*, vol 20, no 7, pp 748-61.

O'Connor, D. and Purves, B. (2009) *Decision-making, personhood and dementia: Exploring the interface*, London: Jessica Kingsley Publishers.

Øderud, T., Landmark, B., Eriksen, S., Fossberg, A.B., Brørs, K.F., Mandal, T.B. and Ausen, D. (2013) 'Exploring the use of GPS for locating persons with dementia', *Assistive Technology Research Series*, vol 33, pp 776-83.

OECD (Organisation for Economic Co-operation and Development) (2015) *Addressing dementia: The OECD response*, OECD Health Policy Studies, Paris: OECD Publishing (http://dx.doi.org/10.1787/9789264231726-en).

OHCHR (Office of the High Commissioner for Human Rights) (2008) *Convention on the Rights of Persons with Disabilities: Advocacy toolkit*, Personal Training Series No 15, Geneva: United Nations (www.ohchr.org/Documents/Publications/AdvocacyTool_en.pdf).

OHCHR (2011) *UN Committee on the Rights of Persons with Disabilities, Consideration of reports submitted by States Parties under Article 35 of the Convention: Concluding observations, Spain, Committee on the Rights of Persons with Disabilities (CRPD)*, 6th Session, at 5, UN Doc CRPD/C/ESP/CO/1, 19-23 September.

OHCHR (2014) *Committee on the Rights of Persons with Disabilities, General Comment No 1, Article 12: Equal Recognition Before the Law*, April, UN Doc. No. CRPD/C/GC/1, adopted at the 11th Session (www.ohchr.org/EN/HRBodies/CRPD/Pages/GC.aspx).

Oliver, M. (1983) *Social work with disabled people*, Basingstoke: Macmillan.

Oliver, M. (1989) 'Disability and dependency: A creation of industrial societies', in L. Barton (ed) *Disability and Dependency*, London: RoutledgeFalmer, pp 7-22.

Oliver, M. (1990) *The politics of disability*, Basingstoke: Macmillan Education.

Oliver, M. (1996) *Understanding disability: From theory to practice*, New York: St Martin's Press.

Oliver, M. (2004) 'The social model in action: If I had a hammer', in C. Barnes and G. Mercer (eds) *Implementing the social model of disability: Theory and research*, Leeds: The Disability Press, pp 18-31.

O'Neill, O. (2002) *Autonomy and trust in bioethics*, Cambridge: Cambridge University Press.

O'Riordan, M. (2011) *Primary care teams – A GP perspective*, Irish College of General Practitioners.

O'Rourke, H.M., Duggleby, W., Fraser, K.D. and Jerke, L. (2015) 'Factors that affect quality of life from the perspective of people with dementia: A metasynthesis', *Journal of the American Geriatrics Society*, vol 63, no 1, pp 24-38.

Orrell, M., Hancock, G., Kumari, D., Liyanage, G. and Woods, B. (2008) 'The needs of people with dementia in care homes: The perspectives of users, staff and family caregivers', *Ageing and Mental Health*, vol 20, no 5, pp 941-51.

O'Shea, E. and Carney, P. (2016) *Dementia paying dividends: A report on the Atlantic philanthropies investment in dementia in Ireland*, Galway: Centre for Economic and Social Research on Dementia, NUI Galway.

O'Shea, E. and O'Reilly, S. (1999) *An action plan for dementia*, Dublin: National Council on Ageing and Older People.

O'Shea, E., Cahill, S. and Pierce, M. (2015) 'Reframing policy for dementia', in K. Walsh, G.M. Carney and A.N. Leime (eds) *Ageing through austerity: Critical perspectives from Ireland*, Bristol: Policy Press, pp 97-112.

O'Sullivan, G. (2013) 'Ethical and effective: Approaches to residential care for people with dementia', *Dementia*, vol 12, no 1, pp 111-21.

Owens, J. (2015) 'Exploring the critiques of the social model of disability: The transformative possibility of Arendt's notion of power', *Sociology of Health and Illness*, vol 37, no 3, pp 385-403.

Palmer, J.L. (2013) 'Preserving personhood of individuals with advanced dementia: Lessons from family caregivers', *Geriatric Nursing*, vol 34, no 3, pp 224-9.

Parker, J. and Penhale, B. (1998) *Forgotten people: Positive approaches to dementia care*, Aldershot: Ashgate.

Parsons, R.J. and Cox, E.O. (1994) *Empowerment-oriented social work practice with the elderly*, Pacific Grove, CA: Brooks/Cole.

Parsons, T. (2015) 'Reminiscence work in four dementia care settings in Ireland: The experience of the person with dementia and the facilitator', Unpublished PhD thesis, Trinity College, Dublin, Ireland.

Peisah, C. and Skladzien, E. (2014) *The use of restraints and psychotropic medications in people with dementia: A report for Alzheimer's Australia*, Paper 38, March.

Perrin, T. and May, H. (2000) *Wellbeing in dementia: An occupational approach for therapists and carers*, Edinburgh: Churchill Livingstone.

Perry, M., Drašković, I., Lucassen, P., Vernooij-Dassen, M., van Achterberg, T. and Rikkert, M.O. (2011) 'Effects of educational interventions on primary dementia care: A systematic review', *International Journal of Geriatric Psychiatry*, vol 26, no 1, pp 1-11.

Phoenix, A. (2008) 'Analysing narrative contexts', in M. Andrews, C. Squire and M. Tamboukou (eds) *Doing narrative research*, London: Sage, pp 64-77.

Pierce, M., Cahill, S., Grey, T. and Dyer, M. (2015) *Research for dementia and home design in Ireland: Looking at new built and retro-fit homes from a universal design approach: Key findings and recommendations 2015*, Centre for Excellence in Universal Design, National Disability Authority (NDA), Ireland.

Pinner, G. and Bouman, W.P. (2003) 'What should we tell people about dementia?', *Advances in Psychiatric Treatment*, vol 9, no 5, pp 335-41.

Pollock, A. (2001) *Designing gardens for people with dementia*, Stirling: Dementia Services Development Centre, University of Stirling.

Pollock, A. and Marshall, M. (2012) *Designing outdoor spaces for people with dementia*, Greenwich, NSW: Hammond Press.

Post, S. (2000) *The moral challenge of Alzheimer's disease: Ethical issues from diagnosis to dying*, Baltimore, MD: Johns Hopkins University.

Pot, A.M. and Petrea, I. (2013) *Improving dementia care worldwide: Ideas and advice on developing and implementing a national dementia plan*, London: Bupa/Alzheimer's Disease International (www.alz.co.uk/sites/default/files/pdfs/global-dementia-plan-report-ENGLISH.pdf).

Pratchett, T. (2008) 'Foreword by Sir Terry Pratchett', in *Dementia out of the shadows*, London: Alzheimer's Society, pp vii-xi (www.mentalhealth.org.uk/file/1202/download?token=LJ-EX684).

Prince, M. (2015) 'Addressing geriatric mental health needs in low income countries', Paper presented at the inaugural Global Brain Health Institute Conference, 8-11 December, Institute Meeting, Havana, Cuba.

Prince, M., Knapp, M., Guerchet, M., McCrone, P., Prina, M., Comas-Herrera, A., Wittenberg, R., Adelaja, B., Hu, B., King, D., Rehill, A. and Salimkumar, D. (2014) *Dementia UK update* (2nd edn), Alzheimer Society.

Quaglio, G., Brand, H. and Dario, C. (2016) 'Fighting dementia in Europe: The time to act is now', *The Lancet Neurology*, vol 15, no 5, pp 452-4.

Quinn, G. (2009) 'Bringing the UN Convention on Rights for Persons with Disabilities to life in Ireland', *British Journal of Learning Disabilities*, vol 37, pp 245-9.

Quinn, G. (2010) 'Personhood and legal capacity. Perspectives on the paradigm shift of Article 12 CRPD', *Conference on Disability and Legal Capacity under the CRPD*, Harvard Law School, Boston, MA, vol 20, pp 3-5.

Quinn, G. (2013a) 'Age: From human deficits to human rights-reflections on a changing field', Paper presented at the launch of the *Human rights and older people policy* paper, Dublin (http://alzheimer. ie/alzheimer/media/SiteMedia/ImageSlider/Fixed/Hr-and-Old-Age-GQfinalX.docx).

Quinn, G. (2013b) 'Rethinking personhood: New directions in legal capacity law and policy', University of British Columbia Centre for Inclusion and Citizenship Conference, Vancouver, 29 April, 4–5 (http://citizenship.sites.olt.ubc.ca/files/2014/07/Gerard_Quinn_s_ Keynote_-_April_29__2011.pdf).

Raeymaekers, P. and Rogers, M.D. (2010) *Improving the quality of life of people with dementia in the EU: A challenge for European society*, Brussels: King Baudouin Foundation.

Ranci, C. and Pavolini, E. (2015) 'Not all that glitters is gold: Long-term care reforms in the last two decades in Europe', *Journal of European Social Policy*, vol 25, no 3, pp 270-85.

Rappe, E. and Topo, P. (2007) 'Contact with outdoor greenery can support competence among people with dementia', *Journal of Housing for the Elderly*, vol 21, pp 229-48.

Redman, M., Taylor, E., Furlong, R., Carney, G. and Greenhill, B. (2012) 'Human rights training: Impact on attitudes and knowledge', *Tizard Learning Disability Review*, vol 17, no 2, pp 80-7.

Rees, G. (2015) 'Dementia-friendly communities: Global initiatives and future directions', Paper presented at 25th Anniversary Celebration, Alzheimer's Disease Association of Singapore.

Rees, G. (2017) 'Global action on dementia', *Australian Journal of Dementia Care*, vol 6, no 4, pp 7-9.

Regulation, L. Act 1871, Dublin: The Stationery Office.

Reichert, E. (2011) *Social work and human rights: A foundation for policy and practice* (2nd edn), New York: Columbia University Press.

Reimer, M.A., Slaughter, S., Donaldson, C., Currie, G. and Eliasziw, M. (2004) 'Special care facility compared with traditional environments for dementia care: A longitudinal study of quality of life', *Journal of the American Geriatrics Society*, vol 52, no 7, pp 1085-92.

Religa, D., Fereshtehnejad, S.M., Cermakova, P., Edlund, A.K., Garcia-Ptacek, S., Granqvist, N. et al (2015) 'SveDem, the Swedish Dementia Registry – A tool for improving the quality of diagnostics, treatment and care of dementia patients in clinical practice', *PLOS One*, vol 10, no 2, e0116538.

Representation Agreement Act (British Columbia) 1996 RSBC Ch. 405.

Retsas, A.P. (1998) 'Survey findings describing the use of physical restraints in nursing homes in Victoria, Australia', *International Journal of Nursing Studies*, vol 35, no 3, pp 184-91.

Revolta, C., Orrell, M. and Spector, A. (2016) 'The biopsychosocial (BPS) model of dementia as a tool for clinical practice. A pilot study', *International Psychogeriatrics*, vol 28, no 7, pp 1079-89.

Robinson, L., Tang, E. and Taylor, J.P. (2015) 'Dementia: Timely diagnosis and early intervention', *BMJ*, vol 350, h3029.

Robinson, L., Brittain, K., Lindsay, S., Jackson, D. and Olivier, P. (2009) 'Keeping in Touch Everyday (KITE) project: Developing assistive technologies with people with dementia and their carers to promote independence', *International Psychogeriatrics*, vol 21, no 3, pp 494-502.

Robinson, L., Hutchings, D., Corner, L., Finch, T., Hughes, J., Brittain, K. and Bond, J. (2007) 'Balancing rights and risks: Conflicting perspectives in the management of wandering in dementia', *Health, Risk & Society*, vol 9, no 4, pp 389-406.

Robinson, L., Gemski, A., Abley, C., Bond, J., Keady, J., Campbell, S. Samsi, K. and Manthorpe, J. (2011) 'The transition to dementia – Individual and family experiences of receiving a diagnosis: A review', *International Psychogeriatrics*, vol 23, no 7, pp 1026-43.

Rochford Brennan, H. (2016) 'My journey with dementia and human rights', Paper presented at launch of Irish Charter of Human Rights for Persons with Dementia, April, Dublin.

Rosenman, L. and Cahill, S. (1989) 'Economic and social costs of Alzheimer's disease, balance', *Journal for the Queensland Association for Mental Health,* vol 1, no 2, pp 18-23.

Russell, C., Middleton, H. and Shanley, C (2008) 'Dying with dementia: The view of family caregivers about quality of life', *Australasian Journal on Ageing*, vol 27, no 2, pp 89-92.

Sabat, S.R. (1994) 'Excess disability and malignant social psychology: A case study of Alzheimer's disease', *Journal of Community & Applied Social Psychology*, vol 4, no 3, pp 157-66.

Sabat, S.R. (2001) *The experience of Alzheimer's disease: Life through a tangled veil*, Oxford and Malden, MA: Blackwell.

Sabat, S.R. (2005) 'Capacity for decision-making in Alzheimer's disease: Selfhood, positioning and semiotic persons', *Australian and New Zealand Journal of Psychiatry*, vol 39, pp 1030-5.

Sabat, S.R. (2011) 'A bio-psycho-social model enhances young adults' understanding of and beliefs about people with Alzheimer's disease: A case study', *Dementia,* vol 11, no 1, pp 95-112.

Sabat, S.R. (2014) 'Understanding people with Alzheimer's disease – A bio psycho-social approach', Paper presented at the Genio Conference, Davenport Hotel, Dublin, December.

Sabat, S.R. and Harré, R. (1992) 'The construction and deconstruction of self in Alzheimer's disease', *Ageing & Society*, vol 12, no 4, pp 443-61.

Samsi, K., Abley, C., Campbell, S., Keady, J., Manthorpe, J., Robinson, L. et al (2014) 'Negotiating a labyrinth: Experiences of assessment and diagnostic journey in cognitive impairment and dementia', *International Journal of Geriatric Psychiatry*, vol 29, no 1, pp 58-67.

Schneider, L.S., Tariot, P.N., Dagerman, K.S., Davis, S.M., Hsiao, J.K., Ismail, M.S. et al (2006) 'Effectiveness of atypical antipsychotic drugs in patients with Alzheimer's disease', *New England Journal of Medicine*, vol 355, no 15, pp 1525-38.

Schulze, M. (2010) *Understanding the UN Convention on the Rights of Persons with Disabilities* (3rd edn), New York: Handicap International.

Scottish Government (2013) *Scotland's national dementia strategy (2013-2016)*, Edinburgh: Scottish Government (www.gov.scot/Resource/0042/00423472.pdf).

Scottish Government (2017) *Scotland's national dementia strategy (2017-2020)*, Edinburgh: Scottish Government (www.gov.scot/Publications/2017/06/7735).

Seanad Éireann Debate, Assisted Decision-Making Capacity Bill (2013) Report and final stages, 15 November, 244(9).

Seanad Éireann debates, 15 December 2015, Vol. 244 No. 9.

Seitz, D.P., Gill, S.S., Austin, P.C., Bell, C.M., Anderson, G.M., Gruneir, A. and Rochon, P.A. (2016) 'Rehabilitation of older adults with dementia after hip fracture', *Journal of the American Geriatrics Society*, vol 64, no 1, pp 47-54.

Shakespeare, T. (2006) *Disability rights and wrongs*, London: Routledge.

Shakespeare, T. (*2014*) *Disability rights and wrongs revisited* (2nd edn), London: Routledge.

Shakespeare, T., Zeilig, H. and Mittler, P. (2017) 'Rights in mind: Thinking differently about dementia and disability', *Dementia*, doi:10.1177/1471301217701506.

SHRC (Scottish Human Rights Commission) (2010) *Care about rights: Human rights and the care of older people*, Information Pack, Glasgow: SHRC.

SHRC (2015) *HRBA/PANEL principles* (http://www.scottishhumanrights.com/rights-in-practice/human-rights-based-approach/).

Silverman, D. (1970) *The theory of organisation: A sociological framework*, London: Heinemann.

Smith, M., Gallagher, M., Wosu, H., Stewart, J., Cree, V.E., Hunter, S. and Evans, S. (*2012*) 'Engaging with involuntary service users in *social work:* Findings from a knowledge exchange project', *British Journal of Social Work*, vol 42, no 8, pp 1460-77.

Solis, M.P. (2014) 'From right to light: A human rights-based approach to universal access to modern energy services', Unpublished PhD thesis, University of Adelaide, Australia.

Sormunen, S., Topo, P., Eloniemi-Sulkava, U., Räikkönen, O. and Sarvimäki, A. (2007) 'Inappropriate treatment of people with dementia in residential and day care', *Ageing and Mental Health*, vol 11, no 3, pp 246-55.

SPCPGOA (Scottish Parliament's Cross-Party Group on Alzheimer's) (2009) *Charter of rights for people with dementia and their carers in Scotland* (http://social.un.org/ageing-working-group/documents/Alzheimer%20Scotland%202.pdf).

Spector, A., Gardner, C. and Orrell, M. (2011) 'The impact of cognitive stimulation therapy groups on people with dementia: Views from participants, their carers and group facilitators', *Aging & Mental Health*, vol 15, no 8, pp 945-9.

Spector, A., Orrell, M. and Goyder, J. (2013) 'A systematic review of staff training interventions to reduce the behavioural and psychological symptoms of dementia', *Ageing Research Review*, vol 12, no 1, pp 354-64.

Spector, A., Hebditch, M., Stoner, C.R. and Gibbor, L. (2016) 'A biopsychosocial vignette for case conceptualization in dementia (VIG-Dem): Development and pilot study', *International Psychogeriatrics*, vol 28, no 9, pp 1471-80.

Spector, A., Orrell, M., Davies, S. and Woods, B. (2000) 'Reality orientation for dementia', *Cochrane Database for Systematic Reviews*, vol 3, CD001119.DOI:10.1002/14651858.CD001119.pub2.

Spector, A., Thorgrimsen, L., Woods, B. and Orrell, M. (2006) *Making a difference: An evidence based group programme to offer cognitive stimulation therapy (CST) to people with dementia*, London: Hawker Publications.

Stainton, T. (2005) 'Empowerment and the architecture of rights based social policy', *Journal of Intellectual Disabilities*, vol 9, no 4, pp 289-98.

Stainton, T. and Clare, I. C. (2012) 'Human rights and intellectual disabilities: An emergent theoretical paradigm?', *Journal of Intellectual Disability Research*, vol 56, no 11, pp 1011-13.

Stokes, G., and Goudie, F. (2002) *The essential dementia care handbook*, Chesterfield: Winslow Press.

Swaffer, K. (2014) 'Dementia: Stigma, language, and dementia-friendly', *Dementia*, vol 13, no 6, pp 709-16.

Swaffer, K. (2016) *What the hell happened to my brain? Living beyond dementia*, London: Jessica Kingsley Publishers.

Sweeting, H. and Gilhooly, M. (1997) 'Dementia and the phenomenon of social death', *Sociology of Health & Illness*, vol 19, no 1, pp 93-117.

Szczepura, A., Wild, D., Khan, A.J., Owen, D.W., Palmer, T., Muhammad, T. et al (2016) 'Antipsychotic prescribing in care homes before and after launch of a national dementia strategy: An observational study in English institutions over a 4-year period', *BMJ Open*, vol 6, no 9, e009882.

Tadd, W., Vanlaere, L. and Gastmans, C. (2010) 'Clarifying the concept of human dignity in the care of the elderly: A dialogue between empirical and philosophical approaches', *Ethical Perspectives – Katholieke Universiteit Leuven*, vol 17, no 2, pp 253-81.

Taft, L.B., Fazio, S., Seman, D. and Stansell, J. (1997) 'A psychosocial model of dementia care: Theoretical and empirical support', *Archives of Psychiatric Nursing*, vol 11, no 1, pp 13-20.

Theurer, K.A. (2012) 'Poster 124 mutual support groups: Social rehabilitation in residential care and in the community', *Archives of Physical Medicine and Rehabilitation*, vol 93, no 10, e50.

Theurer, K.A., Mortenson, B., Stone, R., Suto, M., Timonen, V. and Rozanova, J. (2015) 'The need for a social revolution in residential care', *Journal of Ageing Studies*, vol 35, pp 201-10.

Thomas, C. (2010) 'Medical sociology and disability theory', in G. Scambler and S. Scambler (eds) *New directions in the sociology of chronic and disabling conditions: Assaults on the lifeworld*, New York: Palgrave Macmillan, pp 37-56.

Thomas, C. and Milligan, C. (2015) 'How can and should UK society adjust to dementia?', Joseph Rowntree Viewpoint, York: Joseph Rowntree Foundation.

Thorgrimsen, L., Selwood, A., Spector, A., Royan, L., de Madariaga Lopez, M., Woods, R.T. and Orrell, M. (2003) 'Whose quality of life is it anyway? The validity and reliability of the Quality of Life-Alzheimer's Disease (QoL-AD) scale', *Alzheimer Disease & Associated Disorders*, vol 17, no 4, pp 201-8.

Tilly, J. and Reed, P. (2006) *Falls, wandering, and physical restraints: interventions for residents with dementia in assisted living and nursing homes*. Alzheimer's Association, Chicago, pp 3-11. (https://www.alz.org/national/documents/fallsrestraints_litereview_II.pdf)

Tilly, J. and Rees, G. (2007) *Consumer-directed care: A way to empower consumers*, Alzheimer's Australia, Paper 11.

Timlin, G. and Rysenbry, N. (2010) *Design for dementia: Improving dining and bedroom environments in care homes*, London: Helen Hamlyn Centre, Royal College of Art.

Tobin, J. (2012) *The right to health in international law*, Oxford: Oxford University Press.

Topo, P. (2009) 'Technology studies to meet the needs of people with dementia and their caregivers: A literature review', *Journal of Applied Gerontology*, vol 28, no 1, pp 5-37.

Topo, P., Mäki, O., Saarikalle, K., Clarke, N., Begley, E., Cahill, S. et al (2004) 'Assessment of a music-based multimedia program for people with dementia', *Dementia*, vol 3, no 3, pp 331-50.

Townsend, P. (2006) 'Policies for the aged in the 21st century: More "structured dependency" or the realisation of human rights?', *Ageing & Society*, vol 26, pp 161-79.

Train, G.H., Nurock, S.A., Manela, M., Kitchen, G. and Livingston, G.A. (2005) 'A qualitative study of the experiences of long-term care for residents with dementia, their relatives and staff', *Aging & Mental Health*, vol 9, no 2, pp 119-28.

Travers, C., Lie, D. and Martin Khan, M. (2015) 'Dementia and the population health approach: Promise, pitfalls and progress. An Australian perspective', *Reviews in Clinical Gerontology*, vol 25, pp 60-71.

UK's Human Rights Act (1998) (www.legislation.gov.uk/ukpga/1998/42/contents).

UN (United Nations) (1948) *Universal Declaration of Human Rights (UDHR)*, General Assembly Resolution 217(III), Geneva, Switzerland: UN (www.un.org/en/universal-declaration-human-rights/).

UN (2006) *Convention on the Rights of Persons with Disabilities (CRPD)*, New York: UN DSPD (www.un.org/development/desa/disabilities/convention-on-the-rights-of-persons-with-disabilities.html).

UN (2016) 'DPR of Korea ratifies CRPD, total ratifications 172', New York: UN DSPD (www.un.org/development/desa/disabilities/news/news/democratic-peoples-republic-of-korea-ratifies-crpd-total-ratifications-172.html).

UN enable (2005) *Report of the Ad Hoc Committee on a Comprehensive and Integral International Convention on the Protection and Promotion of the Rights and Dignity of Persons with Disabilities on its fifth session* (www.un.org/esa/socdev/enable/rights/ahc5reporte.htm).

UN enable (2006) *UN Convention on the Human Rights of People with Disabilities Ad Hoc Committee – Daily summary of discussion at the seventh session*, 18 January (www.un.org/esa/socdev/enable/rights/ahc7sum18jan.htm).

UNECE (United Nations Economic Commission for Europe) (2015a) 'Innovative and empowering strategies for care', Policy Brief on Aging, No 15 (www.unece.org/fileadmin/DAM/pau/age/Policy_briefs/ECE-WG.1-21-PB15.pdf).

UNECE (2015b) 'Dignity and non-discrimination for persons with dementia', UNECE policy brief on ageing, No 16 (www.unece.org/population/ageing/policybriefs.html).

UN General Assembly (1979) *Convention on the Elimination of All Forms of Discrimination Against Women*, General Assembly Resolution 34/180, UN Doc A/34/46, 18 December (entered into force 3 September 1981), Article 15.

UN General Assembly (2010) *Follow-up to the Second World Assembly on Ageing*, December, A/65/18 (www.unescap.org/resources/ga-resolution-65182-follow-second-world-assembly-ageing).

UN General Assembly (2011) *Political declaration of the High-level Meeting of the General Assembly on the prevention and control of non-communicable diseases* (www.un.org/ga/search/view_doc.asp?symbol=A/66/L.1).

UPIAS (Union of the Physically Impaired against Segregation) (1976) *Fundamental principles of disability* (http://disability-studies.leeds.ac.uk/files/library/UPIAS-fundamental-principles.pdf).

van Gorp, B. and Vercruysse, T. (2012) 'Frames and counter-frames giving meaning to dementia: A framing analysis of media content', *Social Science & Medicine*, vol 74, no 8, pp 1274-81.

van Hout, H., Vernooij-Dassen, M., Bakker, K., Blom, M. and Grol, R. (2000) 'General practitioners on dementia: Tasks, practices and obstacles', *Patient Education and Counseling*, vol 39, no 2, pp 219-25.

Vassallo, M., Poynter, L., Kwan, J., Sharma, J.C. and Allen, S.C. (2016) 'A prospective observational study of outcomes from rehabilitation of elderly patients with moderate to severe cognitive impairment', *Clinical Rehabilitation*, vol 30, no 9, pp 901-8.

Velasquez, M., Andre, C., Shanks, T., Meyers, S.J. and Meyers, J.M. (2014) *Rights*, Santa Clara, CA: Markkula Center for Applied Ethics (www.scu.edu/ethics/ethics-resources/ethical-decision-making/rights/).

Verbeek, H. (2011) 'Redesigning dementia care: An evaluation of small-scale, homelike care environments', PhD thesis, Maastricht University.

Verbeek, H. (2013) 'Redesigning dementia care: Small scale homelike care environments', Paper presented at Living with Dementia Seminar, Trinity College, Dublin, Ireland, 5 April.

Verbeek, H., van Rossum, E., Zwakhalen, S.M., Kempen, G.I. and Hamers, J.P. (2009) 'Small, homelike care environments for older people with dementia: A literature review', *International Psychogeriatrics*, vol 21, no 2, pp 252-64.

Verdugo, M.A., Navas, P., Gómez, L.E. and Schalock, R L. (2012) 'The concept of quality of life and its role in enhancing human rights in the field of intellectual disability', *Journal of Intellectual Disability Research*, vol 56, no 11, pp 1036-45.

Vernooij-Dassen, M.J., Moniz-Cook, E.D., Woods, R.T., Lepeleire, J.D., Leuschner, A., Zanetti, O. et al (2005) 'Factors affecting timely recognition and diagnosis of dementia across Europe: From awareness to stigma', *International Journal of Geriatric Psychiatry*, vol 20, no 4, pp 377-86.

Vogt, H., Ulvestad, E., Eriksen, T.E. and Getz, L. (2014) 'Getting personal: Can systems medicine integrate scientific and humanistic conceptions of the patient?', *Journal of Evaluation in Clinical Practice*, vol 20, no 6, pp 942-52.

Ward, A. (2015) Abolition of guardianship? "Best interests" versus "best interpretation"', *Scots Law Times*, vol 32, pp 150-4.

Ward-Griffin, C., McWilliam, C.L. and Oudshoorn, A. (2012) 'Relational experiences of family caregivers providing home-based end-of-life care', *Journal of Family Nursing*, vol 18, no 4, pp 491-516.

Wang, W.W. and Moyle, W. (2005) 'Physical restraint use on people with dementia: A review of the literature', *Australian Journal of Advanced Nursing*, vol 22, no 4, p 46.

Welford, C., Murphy, K., Wallace, M. and Casey, D. (2010) 'A concept analysis of autonomy for older people in residential care', *Journal of Clinical Nursing*, vol 19, pp 1226-35.

Welsh, S., Hassiotis, A., O'Mahoney, G. and Deahl, M. (2003) 'Big brother is watching you – The ethical implications of electronic surveillance measures in the elderly with dementia and in adults with learning difficulties', *Aging & Mental Health*, vol 7, no 5, pp 372-5.

Weyerer, S., Schäufele, M. and Hendlmeier, I. (2010) 'Evaluation of special and traditional dementia care in nursing homes: Results from a cross-sectional study in Germany', *International Journal of Geriatric Psychiatry*, vol 25, no 11, pp 1159-67.

WHO (World Health Organization) (1946) *Constitution of WHO: Principles*, Geneva: WHO (www.who.int/about/mission/en/).

WHO (2001) *International classification of functioning, disability and health (ICF)*, Geneva: WHO.

WHO (2002) *World health report 2002: Reducing risks, promoting healthy life*, Geneva: WHO.

WHO (2012) *Dementia: A public health priority*, Geneva: WHO.

WHO (2015a) *Ensuring a human rights-based approach for people living with dementia*, Geneva, Switzerland: WHO (www.ohchr.org/Documents/ Issues/OlderPersons/Dementia/ThematicBrief.pdf).

WHO (2015b) *First WHO ministerial conference on global action against dementia, Meeting report*, 16-17 March, Geneva, Switzerland: WHO (http:// apps.who.int/iris/bitstream/10665/179537/1/9789241509114_eng. pdf).

WHO (2016) *Draft global action plan on the public health response to dementia*, Report by the Director-General, EB 140/28, 23 December (http://apps.who.int/gb/ebwha/pdf_files/EB140/B140_28-en.pdf).

WHO and The World Bank (2011) *World report on disability*, Geneva, WHO and The World Bank.

Wiersma, E.C. and Denton, A. (2016) 'From social network to safety net: Dementia-friendly communities in rural northern Ontario', *Dementia*, vol 15, no 1, pp 51-68.

Williamson, T. (2015) 'Dementia rights and the social model of disability', *Journal of Dementia Care,* vol 23, no 5, pp 12-14.

Wimo, A. (2015) 'The cost of dementia care', Paper delivered at first Dementia Forum X, Stockholm, 18 May.

Wimo, A., Jönsson, L., Bond, J., Prince, M., Winblad, B. and Alzheimer's Disease International (2013) 'The worldwide economic impact of dementia 2010', *Alzheimer's & Dementia*, vol 9, no 1, pp 1-11.

Winblad, B., Amouyel, P., Andrieu, S., Ballard, C., Brayne, C., Brodaty, H. et al (2016) 'Defeating Alzheimer's disease and other dementias: A priority for European science and society', *The Lancet Neurology*, vol 15, no 5, p 455.

Woods, B. (1999) 'Promoting well-being and independence for people with dementia', *International Journal of Geriatric Psychiatry*, vol 14, no 2, pp 97-105.

Woods, B., Spector, A., Jones, C., Orrell, M. and Davies, S. (2005) 'Reminiscence therapy for dementia', *Cochrane Database of Systematic Reviews*, 2: CD001120.DOI:10.1002/14651858.CD001120.pub2.

Woods, R. (2001) 'Discovering the person with Alzheimer's disease: Cognitive emotional and behavioural aspects', *Ageing and Mental Health*, vol 55, suppl 1, S7-16.

World Dementia Council (2014) (https://worlddementiacouncil.org/about-us)

Wortmann, M. (2013) 'Importance of national plans for Alzheimer's disease and dementia', *Alzheimer's Research & Therapy*, vol 5, no 5, p 40.

Wu, Y.T., Fratiglioni, L., Matthews, F.E., Lobo, A., Breteler, M.M., Skoog, I. and Brayne, C. (2016) 'Dementia in Western Europe: Epidemiological evidence and implications for policy making', *The Lancet Neurology*, vol 15, no 1, pp 116-24.

Wübker, A., Zwakhalen, S.M., Challis, D., Suhonen, R., Karlsson, S., Zabalegui, A. et al (2014) 'Costs of care for people with dementia just before and after nursing home placement: Primary data from eight European countries', *The European Journal of Health Economics*, pp 1-19.

Zeisel, J., Silverstein, N.M., Hyde, J., Levkoff, S., Lawton, M.P. and Holmes, W. (2003) 'Environmental correlates to behavioral health outcomes in Alzheimer's special care units', *The Gerontologist*, vol 43, no 5, pp 697-711.

Zimmerman, S., Anderson, W., Brode, S., Jonas, D., Lux, L., Beeber, A. et al (2013) 'Systematic review: Effective characteristics of nursing homes and other residential long term care settings for people with dementia', *Journal of the American Geriatrics Society*, vol 61, no 8, pp 1399-409.

Zwijsen, S.A., Niemeijer, A.R. and Hertogh, C.M. (2011) 'Ethics of using assistive technology in the care for community-dwelling elderly people: An overview of the literature', *Aging & Mental Health*, vol 15, no 4, pp 419-27.

Index

Note: Page numbers in *italics* indicate tables and figures. Page numbers followed by an 'n' refer to end-of-chapter notes.